Published in the UK in 2019 by Rescue Guide

www.rescueguide.co.uk

publishing@rescueguide.co.uk

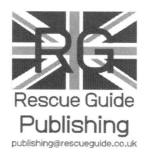

Rescue Guide
Publishing
publishing@rescueguide.co.uk

The information in this guide has been compiled from current best practice, national guidelines and consensus statements from professional bodies; it does not represent any particular organisations standard operating procedures or policies and is intended as guidance only. It is important to work within your organisation's standard operating procedures and your individual scope of practice.

Contents

Introduction

Community First Responders (CFR's) are an important part of the ambulance service's response to emergency medical incidents in the community, often providing early basic life support through early cardiopulmonary resuscitation (CPR) and defibrillation.

Every year in the UK there are over 30,000 out of hospital cardiac arrests (OHCA) in which resuscitation is attempted (BHF, 2014). The importance of providing basic life support quickly following a cardiac arrest cannot be underestimated, as every minute without effective CPR a person's chances of survival reduce by round 7 to 10 percent and brain tissue death starts at around 4 minutes. Early CPR is about saving brain and heart tissue until defibrillation can be carried out, and the more of this we save the more likely our patient is to survive to discharge from hospital.

This book takes the reader through the skills that a CFR may be required to learn and why these skills are important. The foundation of this book is that simple skills save lives. I was not so sure when I first heard the saying; I had seen surgeons doing mind blowing things on TV, and anaesthetists (a word I can never say properly for some reason) cracking someone's chest open at the roadside and restarting their heart. When I became a community first responder though, it all started to make sense. Unfortunately, except in an extremely rare set of circumstances, the surgeon or anaesthetist is never first on scene and somebody has to intervene in those early minutes to ensure that the patient is in a condition that allows the doctors to do what they do. Someone has to keep the blood flowing around the patient's body, otherwise too much damage will have occurred by the time the cavalry arrives.

Being a CFR is not only about CPR though, since becoming a CFR myself around 5 years ago I have attended a range of jobs, some of which required only two skills, reassurance and empathy. Some of the jobs involved mental health issues others involved situations that were not life threatening but the patients were confused and scared. There are also the jobs that can really test your professionalism, the callers who obviously should not have called 999 and those who are abusive when you arrive.

The ability to remain professional in these situations is another important attribute required of a community responder.

Confidentiality is another extremely important part of the role, as much as you trust that your friends and family would never pass on anything you tell them, you simply cannot discuss your patients with anyone other than the patient; their relatives, unless the patient doesn't wish you to do so, and the ambulance crew when they arrive. Breaches of patient confidentiality are a serious matter; after all, if I were the patient I probably would not want everybody knowing about my medical issues.

I have been working in the emergency services as a frontline responder for around 15 years now, mostly responding as part of a team. Despite this experience the first time my pager went off my adrenaline levels went through the roof, the drive was pretty stressful and I almost forgot that as a volunteer I wasn't responding on blue lights and I couldn't understand why traffic wasn't getting out of the way; thankfully I didn't run any reds! This is something that took a while to get used to. Anyway, by the time I arrived my hands were shaking from the stress of the drive and the adrenaline, and I would have been pretty useless had the situation required a steady hand. It seems strange saying thankfully, but thankfully the job just involved a lot of vomit and a patient who was sick but not in any danger, also the ambulance was only about two or three minutes behind me, although it was a long two or three minutes. It was like this for the first three or four jobs, which all came within hours of booking myself available; it was a real eye opener.

The first cardiac arrest I attended was nothing like this though, the training kicked in and I just got on with what needed to be done. The support network kicked in following this incident, and I received multiple welfare calls from the control desk, my team leader and the community resuscitation officer who looked after my area. This is another important part of the system. No matter how long you have been responding for, or how many incidents you have attended; anyone can be affected by stress resulting from the job. You can attend hundreds of cardiac arrests and just one job can trigger something in your mind that you cannot quite shake off.

Ambulance service trusts put in place robust welfare arrangements for their staff and volunteers, but it's not only down to the trust, as responders we should support each other, and it's your fellow responders that often have the greatest understanding of what you are going through.

It's not all doom and gloom though, I have met lots of great people since I started responding and you definitely get the sense that you are really making a difference, and if you make a difference to just one person then surely you have done something worthwhile? Remember, your value is not measured in how much you get paid; as a volunteer you are a valuable part of the chain of survival.

Scope of Practice

Scope of practice outlines what an individual responder is qualified and competent to carry out, it's what they have been trained to do by the ambulance service trust for whom they are going to respond to emergency incidents for. A defined scope of practice is put in place for the protection of the patient and the responder, who runs the risk of legal action should they operate outside of their scope of practice and make their patient's condition worse.

I compare it to someone working on a gas boiler when they are not trained to do so, and there is an explosion, or a DIY enthusiast carrying out structural work on a building and it collapses; the vast majority of people wouldn't attempt either of these so why would anyone risk it with a patient.

Different ambulance service trusts may have different scopes of practice, each trust can decide what level they are going to train their responders to and what types of incident they will be asked to attend.

An example of working outside of your scope of practice would be taking a patient's blood sugar using their own equipment when you are not trained to do so, you can get the patient to do this for you if possible, but you shouldn't do it yourself unless your trust has trained you to.

Consent

Before examining or treating a patient, it is vitally important that you get the patient's permission. A patient can give this consent verbally, so you ask the patient if they mind if you take their pulse and they say you can; or by other means, so you ask the same question and the patient holds out their arm to you.

There may be occasions where a patient's decision to withhold consent may not seem sensible to you as a responder, but unless it is proven that the individual does not have the capacity to make a decision for themselves, then they have the right to refuse.

Capacity

In the vast majority of cases, determining whether your patient has capacity will be straight forward, but there will be cases where it is not quite so straightforward.

Everybody has the legal right to refuse treatment, and even if we believe the decision to be unwise we have to respect it unless it is deemed that the patient does not have the capacity to make such a decision.

The Mental Capacity Act 2005 lays out the rules on deciding whether a person has capacity. There are five key principles contained within the act.

1	A person must be assumed to have capacity unless it is established that they lack capacity.
2	A person is not to be treated as unable to make a decision unless all practicable steps to help them to do so have been taken without success.
3	A person is not to be treated as unable to make a decision merely because they make an unwise decision.
4	An act done or decision made under this Act, for or on behalf of a person who lacks capacity must be done, or made, in their best interests.
5	Before the act is done, or the decision is made, regard must be had to whether the purpose for which it is needed can be as effectively achieved in a way that is less restrictive of the person's rights and freedom of action.

Table 1 - 5 Principles of the Mental Capacity Act 2005

Equipment Checks

There is nothing worse than turning up to a job and finding an important piece of equipment missing, or not working because the batteries have run out. It is frustrating, it looks unprofessional and it can have repercussions for you and your patient.

Taking a small amount of time each week to carry out an equipment check can save a lot of embarrassment and stress later. It is important to check the functionality of your equipment, use by dates on consumables especially drugs such as aspirin, and test dates on oxygen or Entonox cylinders.

These checks should be recorded, as if anything does go wrong, and you happen to end up giving evidence at a coroner's court hearing, you will have the evidence to back you up.

Personal Equipment

In terms of medical equipment, firstly it is important that you only carry what you are trained and competent to use. Secondly for the safety of you and your patient it is also critical that the equipment you are using has been approved by your trust and has been supplied by an approved supplier; should something go wrong this is the kind of thing that will be looked at in any subsequent investigation, which may ultimately lead all the way to a coroners court.

There are however certain items of equipment that may not supplied by the trust but can be useful to carry; items such as head torches, warm blankets, sugary drinks for those with low blood sugar (if your trust allows this), and maps (Ordnance Survey, Street Maps etc.).

Dynamic Risk Assessment

From the minute your pager goes off, to the time that you arrive back at home you should be going through a process of identifying hazards and implementing control measures; this process is known as dynamic risk assessment, or DRA.

Whatever we are doing and wherever we are, the environment around us is constantly changing. At an emergency incident the rate at which this change occurs can increase significantly, hazards that we are aware of can change and new hazards can appear. The process of dynamic risk assessment involves being aware of these hazards, monitoring them and putting control measures in place.

Even running to the car is not without risk; uneven or wet surfaces, ice and snow, potholes, open drain covers, and traffic all present a risk. Once in your vehicle, I would say that the risk increases significantly; if your mind is on what you can expect at the incident rather than the road it is all too easy to make a mistake, and it is not just you, other motorists are a hazard. Weather conditions and the condition of the road surface can also catch out the unwary driver.

The process does not stop at identifying hazards though; it is no good spotting the hazard if you do not do anything about it. Some common examples of control measures include:

- Slowing down in wet weather;
- Slowing down and moving over to avoid potholes;
- Giving extra room to horse riders and cyclists, and
- Ensuring your exit route is kept clear at the scene of an incident.

Driving to the Scene

When driving to the scene it is very easy to concentrate on what might be waiting for you when you arrive, and the feeling that you need to get there as fast as is humanly possible can be difficult to shake off; this is only natural. What you need to focus on is your driving, and the responder's biggest enemy when driving is the red mist. Getting frustrated with other drivers is all too easy, especially when you are responding to a life-threatening emergency, but it is important to remember that they do not know that you are responding to a medical emergency, and the red mist can cause people to take unnecessary risks. Exceeding the speed limit and taking that risky overtake often makes surprisingly little difference to your overall journey time; anyone who commutes on a busy motorway during rush hour will attest to the fact that you often reach your junction at the same time as the idiot who overtook you earlier at ninety.

Now, I am aware that some responder schemes around the UK do respond on blue lights, and that is down to the individual trust to decide. The vast majority of schemes choose not to allow their responders to drive on blue lights, and this is perfectly understandable as the issues surrounding the cost of supplying a suitable vehicle, insurance and the vast training implications can be difficult to manage.

It is also worth remembering that driving on blue lights comes with great responsibility, and should you cause an accident you are open to prosecution just as any other driver is, and you are expected to maintain a far higher standard.

A big part of blue light driving is not treating red traffic lights as a give way or speeding past vehicles on the wrong side of the road, it's more about identifying and responding to hazards, anticipation of potential problems ahead, and forward planning. For example if you are following a bus and passengers begin to stand up then you can reasonably assume that the bus is approaching a stop and will be pulling over to the left shortly. Other examples include:

- Bins placed at the side of the road are a sign that there may be slow moving or stationary refuse vehicles in the road;
- Mud on the road may indicate the presence of slow moving agricultural vehicles or construction traffic, and
- Horse poo may indicate that this is a route used by horse riders!

Switch between what is happening in front of you and what is going on in the distance, this allows you to plan ahead and anticipate problems. When driving on the motorway or a dual carriageway you can generally predict that a vehicle is going to overtake if it is catching up with the vehicle in front.

Finally, always assume that other drivers are going to pull out on you or make mistakes, and on narrow roads always drive as if there is something around the corner; that way you will always be ready to react to whatever happens.

Electronic Devices

Whether driving on blue lights or observing normal road rules, operating electronic devices while driving is not only illegal, it is dangerous as well. As a solo responder, pulling over in a safe place to reply to a radio message; send a reply on your pager or type an address into your sat nav is a must. it's better for you and the patient to do this and arrive safely, than it is not to arrive at all.

Remember, hands free phones should be set up prior to your journey, and the law on using mobile communications devices includes their use when stationary in traffic or at traffic lights. At the time of writing, the penalty for using a handheld mobile phone whilst driving is 6 penalty points and a £200 fine, meaning that if you get caught twice you will probably be facing a driving ban, and this can also result in the loss of your primary source of income. The risks far outweigh the benefits.

Another point to remember is visibility. Placing a device in a position on your windscreen that affects your forward visibility is not only dangerous, it is also an offence punishable by three penalty points; this includes satellite navigation and other electronic devices, not just mobile phones.

Arrival on Scene

The first thing to consider when arriving on scene is parking, it is important to leave space for an ambulance and park legally in a safe place. Some trusts recommend putting your hazard lights on to make it easier for the oncoming crews to identify the location of the incident, although this often relies on the crews being informed that a responder has also been dispatched to the incident.

From here it is time to start assessing the scene; is the door already open, are there any hazards such as grumpy looking dogs between you and the door; often if something just doesn't feel right then it isn't. If the door is closed, knock and wait to be invited in, if it is open then shout through and identify yourself. If there is no answer, check any windows for signs of an unconscious patient, if there are no signs and you cannot gain access then contact your control room for further advice or backup. Many fire and rescue services can gain entry to a property without causing significant damage or sometimes no damage at all.

Scene Safety and Assessment

In terms of safety at incidents, there is a good hierarchy to follow (shamelessly stolen from the water rescue world), and that is self; team; victim. In the context of medical emergencies this may be better worded as self; team; patient. Look after your own safety first, after all you do not want to become a patient yourself, then the safety of your team i.e. ambulance crews and other responders, and then the patient. If you see something dangerous do not be afraid to speak up.

Scene assessment begins the minute you exit your vehicle, this is where you switch your brain from driving mode to incident mode. The overwhelming urge when arriving on scene can be to find and help the patient; it's a natural instinct, particularly for those who have signed up to help others. The problem with rushing in and becoming task focussed is that you don't see the potential hazards at or around the scene, potentially putting you at risk of becoming a second casualty and making the overall situation worse; which is the complete opposite of the reason that you are there in the first place.

The classic example would be the scene at which there are two or more patients and no apparent reason as to why they are incapacitated. This should immediately start alarm bells ringing for the first responder, and as difficult as it is to resist the urge to rush in and help, the best course of action is to pause and assess the scene thoroughly before acting. The saying "fools rush in" is very appropriate when it comes to scene assessment.

Once you have sized up the scene you can put in any control measures required, providing it is safe to do so. Examples of this would be turning off an electrical appliance at the socket or turning off a gas fire.

Hazards, Risk and Control Measures

When carrying out a dynamic risk assessment it is important to have an understanding of the terms hazard, risk and control measure.

A hazard is something with the potential to cause harm, based on that, I think you would agree that a lion is a hazard. So the risk when you open the door and are faced with a lion is that it attacks you and has you for lunch, and the chances of this happening if you walk into a room with a hungry lion are pretty high.

To prevent the lion from snacking on us we need to put control measures in place if they are not already. A control measure is something we put in place to eliminate or reduce the risk of harm occurring as the result of a hazard. For example, if I put the lion in a cage, or move it into another room then it no longer poses a risk; it is also worth asking yourself whether you can complete your task without going into the room in the first place.

When deciding on a control measure you should start with the one that eliminates the hazard altogether, if that is not possible then you try the one that reduces the likelihood or harm occurring the most and so on. Eventually you will reach a point where the risks outweigh the benefits, for example, there is a small chance you may save your patient, but the lion will definitely eat you, this is known as benefit versus risk. (Thankfully, the chances of coming across a lion while responding are remote!)

A good mnemonic to remember when looking at control measures is ERIC PD:

E	**Eliminate**	An example of this would be shutting an overly protective dog in another room therefore eliminating the hazard.
R	**Reduce**	When driving in the rain we reduce our speed to reduce the likelihood of an accident occurring.
I	**Isolate**	Putting a physical barrier between you and the hazard.
C	**Control**	Safe systems of work for example waiting for the police to arrive where there is a risk of violence.
P	**PPE**	Providing PPE to protect us from the hazard, an example of this is nitrile gloves.
D	**Discipline**	Ensuring that policies and procedures are strictly adhered to.

ERIC PD takes a stepwise approach to the selection of control measures, starting with the most preferable and working down in order.

Hazards in the Home

It is important to remember that your DRA continues when you enter the property, just because a situation seems routine does not mean that there are no hazards present. In the home, you will find utilities such as gas and electricity, hostile occupiers and unfriendly animals as I once found out, almost to my cost when I was chased down a driveway by a rather angry German shepherd; fortunately, I made it to the gate before he did. It is amazing how fast you can run with a land shark on your tail.

A good example of a potential hazard in the home is carbon monoxide. Carbon monoxide is a big hazard, and several patients all presenting with the same symptoms in the same property would certainly set alarm bells ringing for me.

Hazards in the Workplace

Emergencies in the workplace often present the greatest number of hazards, and often put the responder at the greatest risk. You may be faced with industrial machinery, heavy goods vehicles, forklift trucks and hazardous materials; fortunately, you should also have members of staff to guide you, but it is important not to put yourself at risk.

Remember that your safety and that of your patient is paramount, if you are not happy with a situation then you should ask staff to close off an area or stop what they are doing if it affects the safety of you and your patient. If this is not possible, consider whether it is safe to move your patient to another part of the site.

High visibility vests or jackets should be worn in the workplace, as well as any other protective equipment that may be required as part of the safe system of work or risk assessment for the premises, such as ear or eye protection.

SAFETY NOTE:
ALWAYS follow the instructions of on-site personnel and follow **ALL** posted health and safety rules including eye and ear protection.

Hazards Outdoors

When responding to emergencies outdoors there are numerous hazards, and they can differ greatly from those you will find in the home or the workplace, particularly where the incident involves the road network. Moving traffic is the one of the biggest hazards you are likely to face as a responder, particularly as you do not have the protection of a high visibility vehicle with blue lights, although from experience I can tell you, even that is no guarantee.

When parking at the roadside it is a good idea to put your hazard warning lights on, particularly at night. Make yourself visible by wearing your high visibility vest or jacket and when working on or near a road be aware that hazard warning lights and high visibility clothing are no guarantee that other drivers will spot you, it is important to keep yourself safe from moving traffic and you should never take any unnecessary risks.

In the winter months, it is important to remember that not only can your patient become hypothermic; you can suffer the effects of the cold yourself. It is important to carry warm clothing in your vehicle, as the colder you get and the more you shiver you will begin to lose your fine motor skills. Trying to carry out tasks when the adrenaline is flowing and you are freezing cold is a bit like trying to tie your shoelaces with boxing gloves on.

SAFETY NOTE:
ALWAYS wear a high visibility jacket when working on or near a road.

Infection Control

Good hygiene is very important, for your own safety and that of your patient. As part of your role you will attend to patients who are suffering from a range of conditions, some of which will be contagious others will not be; for your safety it is important to protect yourself.

Some patients you treat may be immunosuppressed (weak immune system) and more susceptible to illness, for example, a cancer patient undergoing chemotherapy will be more susceptible to picking up illnesses and their body's ability to fight them off will be greatly reduced. Where this is the case, it is important to protect your patient from any illnesses you may have picked up.

The foundation of infection control is good personal hygiene, hand washing, and the use of hand gels. Where bodily fluids such as blood come into contact with your clothes you should change them at the earliest opportunity, and certainly before seeing another patient; I tend to carry a spare shirt in the car just in case.

When washing your hands you should pay particular attention to the areas where bacteria can hide, such as underneath the fingernails and in between the fingers, and don't forget your wrists and forearms, after all there is no magic barrier stopping germs from passing your wrists.

The wearing of personal items such as watches should be avoided as they could potentially harbour harmful bacteria. Ideally you should be bare from the elbows down.

Infection control does not stop with the CFR, it is important that the same level of hygiene control be maintained with your equipment, particularly where bodily fluids are spilt on it. Approved wipes available from your trust can be used to clean off blood and other bodily fluids, and it is vital that you wear disposable gloves while doing this.

Safeguarding

As a community first responder, you have a duty of care over your patients and this duty includes the reporting of safeguarding issues. My biggest worry when first introduced to safeguarding was knowing what to report, and what happens if I report something and there turns out to be a completely innocent explanation.

When I really thought about it though, I came to the realisation that it was better to report something and be wrong, than not to report something and be right. There have been several high profile cases where suspected abuse has gone unreported, and children have slipped through the net with tragic consequences. These situations could be avoided if people take action and report things that just do not seem right.

Statistically the main forms of abuse in the UK are:

- Physical;
- Neglect;
- Financial;
- Psychological, and
- Sexual.

Exploitation is another safeguarding issue to be aware of. Exploitation includes modern slavery; human trafficking; radicalisation of vulnerable people and forced labour. This may or may not be for the personal gain of the individual(s) involved.

People with learning difficulties, or those who are ill, old or infirm are more at risk of abuse, but it is important to remember that anyone can be abused, and anyone can be an abuser.

Recognising abuse can be difficult as abusers can become adept at covering up what they are doing. Signs may include frequent or unexplained injuries; signs of malnutrition; changes in behaviour when the abuser is present, or bruising, burns and other injuries inconsistent with an accident.

Your trust will have a specific safeguarding policy in place including reporting procedures. It is a good idea to familiarise yourself with these policies, and have the reporting procedure in your kit bag or written down in a notebook. If you are unsure, you can always speak to the ambulance crew when they arrive.

> Note:
> Remember; never put yourself in any danger. Your safety comes first.

Advance Decisions

When delivering training to CFR's, advance decisions or advanced directives are a subject that often causes plenty of conversation, as well as some concern. The biggest concerns are what happens if the paperwork is not available and the responder treats or does not treat the patient, especially under pressure from relatives, or the scenario where one relative wants you to treat but another does not.

In the UK, we all have the right to refuse treatment if we have the mental capacity to do so. The advance decision, sometimes known as a living will is a decision than can be made now, to refuse certain types of treatment in the future. The document must outline all of the treatments that are being refused, and there may be some situations in which the patient wants to refuse treatment and others where they wish to be treated. The treatment being refused may include CPR or assisted ventilation.

An advanced decision must list the treatments and situations that are to be refused; it must be written down and signed by both the person making the decision and a witness. In order to be legally binding the decision must comply with the Mental Capacity act 2005, it must apply to the present situation, and it must be valid. When the decision meets these requirements then it cannot be overruled by family members or anyone else, regardless of their intentions.

The patient can choose who gets to see the decision, but it is important that it is available and can be produced quickly if the patient requires treatment that has been refused. If this treatment is lifesaving, such as CPR or defibrillation the document must be signed by a witness, it must also include a statement outlining the decision to refuse treatment even if that refusal means that the patient could die.

The decision to refuse CPR may also be made and communicated to the medical team. This is known as a DNACPR (do not attempt CPR) order or decision. If the patient makes it clear to the medical team that they do not wish to have CPR then this will be entered into their medical records and recorded on a form. These orders are not permanent, and the patient has the right to change their mind at any point.

Validity of an Advance Decision
In order to be deemed as valid the decision must: • Specify clearly what treatments are being refused; • Explain the situations in which treatment is being refused; • Be signed by the patient; • If lifesaving treatment is being refused, be signed by a witness; • Be made without outside influence (i.e. under pressure from others); **The patient making the decision must be over 18 years of age and have the capacity to make the decision; they must also have not done anything since making the decision stating that they have changed their mind.**

**DO NOT ATTEMPT
CARDIOPULMONARY RESUSCITATION (DNACPR)**
Adults aged 16 years and over. In the event of cardiac or respiratory
arrest do not attempt cardiopulmonary resuscitation (CPR).
All other appropriate treatment and care will be provided.

**NHS
East of England**

DO NOT PHOTOCOPY

Name:	(OR USE ADDRESSOGRAPH)	**ORIGINAL** PATIENT COPY TO STAY WITH PATIENT
Address:		
	Postcode:	**Date of DNACPR order:**
NHS number:	Date of birth:	

REASON FOR DNACPR DECISION (tick one or more boxes and provide further information)

☐ CPR is unlikely to be successful (i.e. medically futile) because:

☐ Successful CPR is likely to result in a length and quality of life not in the best interests of the patient because:

☐ Patient does not want to be resuscitated as evidenced by:

RECORD OF DISCUSSION OF DECISION (tick each box and provide further information)

Discussed with the patient / Lasting Power of Attorney (welfare)? Yes ☐ No ☐
If 'yes' record content of discussion. If 'no' say why not discussed.

Discussed with relatives / carers / others? Yes ☐ No ☐
If 'yes' record name, relationship to patient and content of discussion. If 'no' say why not discussed.

Discussed with other members of the health care team? Yes ☐ No ☐
If 'yes' record name, role and content of discussion. If 'no' say why not discussed.

Is DNACPR decision indefinite? Yes ☐ No ☐ If 'no' specify review date:

HEALTHCARE PROFESSIONAL COMPLETING THIS DNACPR ORDER				
Name:		Signature:		
Position:		Date:		Time:

REVIEW AND ENDORSEMENT BY RESPONSIBLE SENIOR CLINICIAN				
Name:		Signature:		
Position:		Date:		Time:

Figure 1 - Example of a DNACPR Form

Anatomy

INTERNAL STRUCTURE OF THE HUMAN BODY

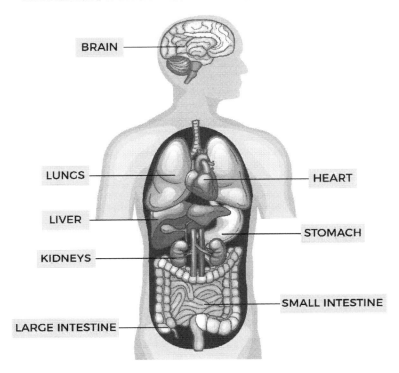

BRAIN

LUNGS

HEART

LIVER

STOMACH

KIDNEYS

SMALL INTESTINE

LARGE INTESTINE

Figure 2 - Major Organs

Musculoskeletal System

The Musculoskeletal system is the reason that we are not simply a pile of human tissue lying on the floor; it is the framework that gives our body its shape, and it protects our vital organs. Attached to the framework by tendons are the muscles that allow us to move.

Muscle

There are three types of muscle in the human body:

- Skeletal, voluntary and reflex muscles;
- Involuntary muscles, and
- Cardiac (Heart) muscle.

These muscles control certain functions and allow us to move and pump blood around the body. Some we have control over (voluntary), and others react without conscious thought (involuntary/cardiac muscle).

Muscular injuries can be painful and cause the patient difficulties, but they are rarely life threatening; with the exception of cardiac muscle of course!

Bones

The adult body has 206 bones. As well as keeping us upright and protecting our vital organs, the bones have other functions such as producing blood in the bone marrow and storing salts and other minerals.

Our bones are categorised into five types:

Long Bones	Femur (Thigh); Radius (Forearm)
Short Bones	Carpals in the wrist
Irregular Bones	Vertebrae (Spinal column)
Flat Bones	Bones in the skull; Sternum
Sesamoid Bones	Patella (Kneecap)

Table 2 – Categories of Bone

The outside of a bone is hard, consisting of a dense layer of bone cells, which gives the bone its strength. The inside consists of spongy bone tissue. Fracturing a bone can be painful and debilitating for the patient, and certain fractures such as pelvic fractures, long bones, ribs and skull can be life threatening. Because of the force required to break a bone, other injuries are usually present.

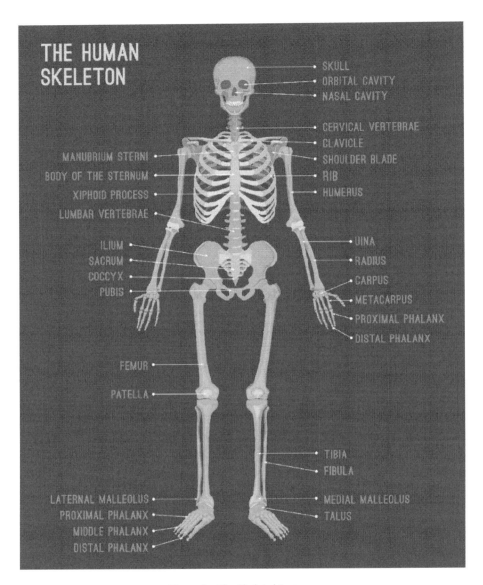

Figure 3 - The Skeletal System

Circulatory System

The circulatory system is the body's transport network, transporting oxygen, nutrients and waste products around the body. I often compare it to our road network, the body's cells are the consumers, the various organs and glands are the producers, the veins and arteries are the roads and the blood is the vehicle that delivers goods and takes away waste products for disposal. As with the road network, blockages (clots) cause issues; if waste products are not collected they build up causing issues, and if there are not enough vehicles to deliver goods (low blood volume) then the consumers (cells) will be unable to function properly. Thankfully, the average person's circulatory system is not constantly blocked and full of potholes!

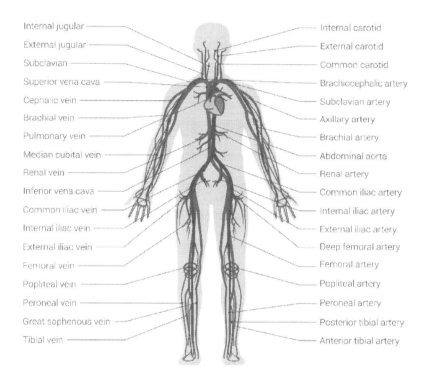

Figure 4 - Circulatory System

Arteries, with the exception of the pulmonary artery, carry oxygenated blood from the heart around the body. The pulmonary artery carries de-oxygenated blood to the lungs to exchange carbon dioxide for oxygen.

Veins do the opposite, with the exception of the pulmonary vein. The veins carry de-oxygenated blood back to the heart from where it is pumped into the lungs. The pulmonary vein carries oxygenated blood back to the heart for distribution throughout the body.

The blood is distributed by the heart at a rate controlled by the brain and the rate is dependent on demands from the body, for example if you are at rest then your muscles do not require as much oxygen, so your heart rate will be lower than when you are exercising and there is increased demand from the muscles.

Respiratory System

The respiratory system is responsible for gas exchange between oxygen and carbon dioxide and maintaining the body's acid base. The body's cells require oxygen in order for metabolism to take place. Metabolism is the process through which the body grows and functions, and the waste products from this process includes carbon dioxide.

The main components in this system are the lungs and the air passages.

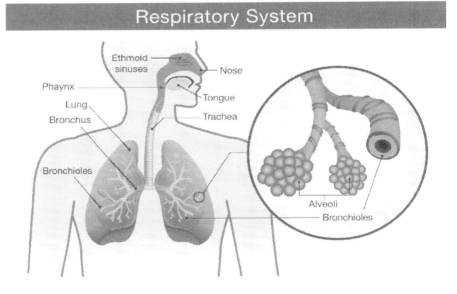

Figure 5 - Respiratory System

From the trachea, the air flows through the left and right bronchus into the bronchioles and then the alveoli. It is in the alveoli where gas exchange takes place and carbon dioxide in the blood is replaced with oxygen. The carbon dioxide is then disposed of when we breathe out.

Digestive System

The digestive system is concerned with getting nutrients into the body and getting rid of any waste products. The process of digestion breaks down the food that we eat into the chemicals that our body needs in order to function. These substances are then absorbed into the blood stream in order to be transported around the body to where they are needed. Any waste products are excreted via the intestinal tract.

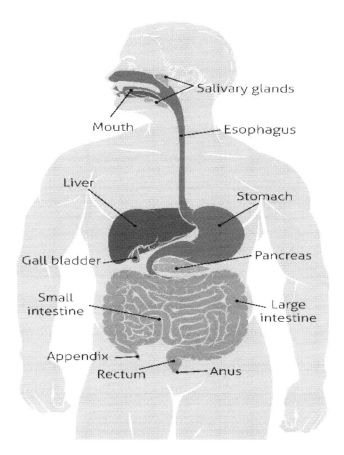

Figure 6 - Digestive System

Nervous System

The nervous system is very complex and consists of the brain, spinal cord and a network of nerves. In basic terms, our senses detect changes in the environment, both internal and external; these are communicated to the brain, which then decides how to react. Once the decision has been made, signals will be sent to the appropriate cells. An example of this was discussed in the previous chapter in which the brain increases the heart rate in response to growing demand for oxygen from the muscles during exercise.

Endocrine System

There are three main components in the endocrine system; these are glands, hormones and receptors. Each of the glands release hormones that have specific purposes, for example the pancreas contains cells that produce glucagon, the hormone that converts glycogen into glucose.

Hormones are transported around the body in the bloodstream. When they reach their destination i.e. an organ, they stick to receptor cells, and these processes cause physiological changes to take place.

Examples of glands in the body include:

Thyroid Gland	Stores and produces hormones that help to regulate blood pressure, metabolic rate, heart rate and body temperature.
Adrenal Glands	Found just above the kidney the adrenal glands produce hormones that help maintain fluid balance, regulate stress resistance, metabolism and produce fight or flight hormones.
The Pancreas	The pancreas secretes digestive enzymes into the small intestine, produces glucagon, which breaks down glycogen into glucose, and also plays a role in the immune system/
The Pineal Gland	Located in the brain, the pineal gland produces melatonin, which plays a part in regulating sleep cycles, reproduction, body temperature and cardiovascular function.

Table 3 - Examples of Glands

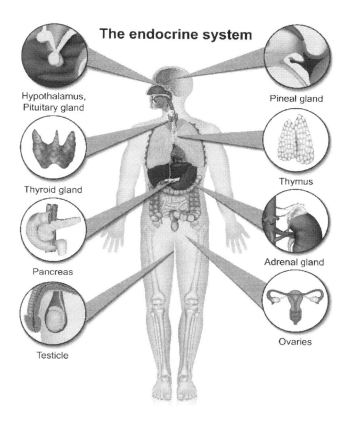

Figure 7 - The Endocrine System

Primary Survey

The primary survey is where we ensure that the important stuff is all in order, the basic faculties that keep us alive. Firstly as we approach our patient we check their level of response; are they fully **alert** and responsive, do they respond to your **voice** but make no reply or groan when you speak to them, do they respond only to **pain**ful stimuli, or are you getting no response whatsoever **(unconscious or unresponsive)**. What you have done in doing this is utilised the AVPU scale.

A	V	P	U
The patient is alert and responsive	The patient responds to your voice	The patient responds to painful stimuli only	The patient is unresponsive (or unconscious)

Table 4 - AVPU Scale

Now we need to check the vitals, we need to know that the patient is not losing blood, that they have a patent airway and they are breathing, and that their blood is circulating in order to carry oxygen and nutrients to their vital organs. We do this in a particular order, starting with major bleeding **(catastrophic haemorrhage)**; after all, there is no point in attempting CPR if there is no blood to pump around the body (you wouldn't attempt to pump a tyre up with holes in it would you). After we have checked for and dealt with any leaks we need to ensure that the patient has an **airway** so that they can get oxygen to their lungs and into the blood stream, we also need to check whether they are **breathing** in the oxygen for themselves, or whether we need to do this for them. Finally, we need to make sure that this oxygenated blood is circulating around the body **(Circulation)**.

Now we have checked for the vitals, providing that these are all present and correct, there are a couple of other checks that form part of our primary survey, the first being **disability.**

In this context, when referring to disability we are referring to neurological deficit i.e. is their brain functioning as it should be. There are numerous reasons why it may not be, for example they may have suffered a stroke or a head injury, both of which can be life threatening.

The final check in our primary survey is **exposure** to the **environment** and how this may be affecting the patient e.g. is the patient becoming hypothermic.

When we put all of this together and add in our scene assessment, we have DR C ABC DE.

For trauma incidents we add an extra 'C' to DR C ABCDE, it is just a little one and it comes after the A. Where we suspect that the patient may have injured their c-spine, we will consider it when managing their airway. To cover this we have DR C A(c)BCDE.

Instead of a head tilt chin lift, a jaw thrust should be carried out on a patient with a suspected c-spine injury; this is to avoid unnecessary movement of the neck.

D	R	C	A	B	C	D	E
Danger	Response	Catastrophic Haemorrhage	Airway	Breathing	Circulation	Disability	Exposure/Environment

Table 5 - DR C ABCDE

KEY POINT:
For non-trauma patients a head tilt chin lift should be carried out.
For trauma patients a jaw thrust should be used.

Cardiopulmonary Resuscitation

If breathing and circulation are not present then we need to take over these functions for the patient, this is known as cardiopulmonary resuscitation or CPR. By carrying out CPR, we are breathing for the patient and compressing their chest in order to compress the heart and pump oxygenated blood around the body. In doing this, we are attempting to circulate oxygenated blood to the heart and brain in order to keep them alive. After several minutes without oxygen, heart and brain tissue begins to die, the more of this tissue that dies the lower the chance of survival, and even if we can get their heart back into normal sinus rhythm on scene, if too much brain or heart muscle tissue has died, they may not survive to discharge from hospital.

The key to good CPR is high quality chest compressions, too shallow and you will not effectively compress the heart, if you do not fully release then you are not allowing adequate blood flow back into the heart. The rate is also important, too slow and you do not build up enough pressure in the system for adequate perfusion (oxygenated blood entering the tissue) to take place, to quick and you are not pumping the blood around the system effectively.

What tends to happen is people start too quickly, then as they become tired they slow down to a good rate and then as they become even more tired the rate becomes too slow. It's a bit like a long distance race, particularly when you are on your own, you need to pace yourself and try to maintain a steady constant rhythm of between 100 and 120 per minute; I have always found that some of the metronome apps available for smart phones can really help with this.

It is, for obvious reasons, far easier to maintain high quality chest compressions with two or more responders by rotating the person on the chest (the person carrying out chest compressions). In this scenario one person can manage the patient's airway, supplementary oxygen and give breaths while the other does chest compressions, they can then rotate every 2 to 3 cycles to avoid fatigue.

Another point to consider is 360° access to the patient. Unfortunately patients rarely collapse in wide-open spaces, it is often down the side of the bed or behind a sofa and even whilst they are on the toilet. Where possible, taking into account your own capabilities, you should attempt to move the patient into the open where 360 degree access to the patient is available, this will make the whole process of resuscitation far easier. If you cannot move the patient alone then you should attempt CPR and wait for another responder or the ambulance crew to arrive.

Chest Compressions

The first thing is hand position and the easiest way to get this right is to aim for the breastbone (sternum).

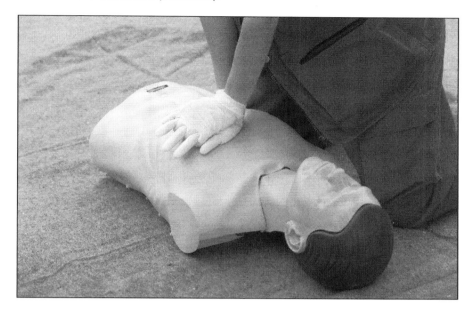

Figure 8 - Hand Position

Place the palm of your hand on the breastbone and the other hand on top with the fingers interlocked as shown. Kneel down close enough to the patient so that when your arms are locked your shoulders are above the centre of chest; locking your arms and positioning yourself close enough means that you are using your bodyweight to compress the chest rather than the muscles in your arms, this is far more affective and reduces fatigue.

Good quality chest compressions are the key to good quality CPR. The key to quality chest compression is depth, rate and full release. Each should be approximately a third of the depth of the chest and you should release fully, this allows blood to fill the heart ready for the next compression.

The rate should be around 100 to 120 per minute; a good way to measure this is one of the many metronome apps available on smartphones. If you prefer you purchase a digital metronome, but the apps can be downloaded for free. Some people prefer to use a song such as Nellie the Elephant, and there was of course the famous 'stayin alive' advert featuring ex footballer turned actor Vinnie Jones; I even know some people who use Run DMC Walk his way!

Respirations

After each set of 30 chest compressions, you should give your patient two breaths, by doing so you are giving your patient the oxygen that you normally breathe out into the atmosphere. The air in the atmosphere consists of around 21% Oxygen and the air that we breathe out consists of around 16% Oxygen, so that leaves plenty for the patient.

There are a couple of things to remember when giving breaths; firstly, you are not trying to blow up a balloon; think about how you breath normally when breathing into your patient, if you over inflate the lungs then some of the air will make its way into the stomach and you run the risk of your patient vomiting. The second thing to remember is infection control; a pocket mask or facemask should be used as the one-way valve will protect you if your patient does vomit.

You may carry and be trained to use a bag valve and mask, the problems with this as a solo responder is that it can be difficult to get a good seal and compress the bag at the same time, and as such it is preferable as a solo responder to use a pocket mask until assistance arrives. The same rule applies when using a pocket mask, don't over-inflate, you don't need to compress the bag like you are trying to squeeze water from a sponge, a thumb and index finger will suffice.

If your two breaths are ineffective, do not waste time trying two more. The time in which your hands are off the patient's chest should be reduced to a minimum. All the time in which you are not carrying out chest compressions the patient's blood pressure is reducing, and this pressure is important in ensuring that the oxygenated blood can penetrate the tissues (perfusion).

Normally when carrying out CPR you will give 30 chest compressions followed by two breaths, the exceptions to this are drowning and children. With drowning cases and children, you should give 5 rescue breaths first.

SAFETY POINT:

If you are using supplementary oxygen and your patient has collapsed in front of the fire, where possible you should turn the fire off. If this is not possible, you **MUST** keep your oxygen cylinder and mask away from the fire.

Pit Crew CPR

Based around the formula one pit stop, pit crew CPR is a structured way of carrying out basic life support on a patient when there are multiple responders present.

The idea is that each responder has a defined role to focus on and taking away the pressure of juggling multiple roles allows each responder to carry out their role to the best of their abilities.

Pit crew CPR also helps to remove the fatigue element of CPR by rotating the responders who are carrying out chest compressions allowing them to rest every 2 minutes or 2 cycles.

The team consists of an airway manager who will be responsible for maintain the patient's airway and giving breaths, or ventilating using a bag valve and mask (BVM). They will also be responsible for pressing the button on the defibrillator to deliver a shock, as they are the ones who have control of the oxygen and can safely remove it before delivering the shock.

The two people on chest compressions will also act as airway assistant, so whoever is not carrying out chest compressions can use a two handed grip to get and effective seal on the mask of the BVM, while the airway manager compresses the bag; they can also pass equipment.

The team leader will record patient observations and manage the rotation of chest compressions; they will also monitor the welfare of the team looking for signs of stress and fatigue.

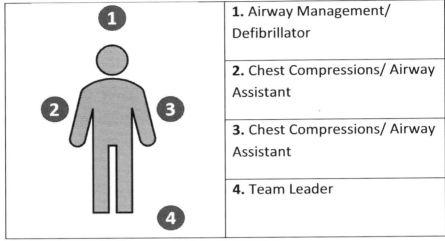

	1. Airway Management/ Defibrillator
	2. Chest Compressions/ Airway Assistant
	3. Chest Compressions/ Airway Assistant
	4. Team Leader

Table 6 - Pit Crew CPR

A key benefit of pit crew CPR is that it allows people to become task focussed, in fact, it is encouraged. Individuals have their own tasks to focus on, often meaning that each task is performed to the very best of the individual's ability. The team leader having an overview of the whole scene means that not everyone else needs to.

Defibrillation

Automatic external defibrillators (AED) are becoming an increasingly common sight in town centres and other public places; they are simple to use and significantly increase the chances of survival for someone in cardiac arrest.

There is often some confusion as to what a cardiac arrest actually is. It is sometimes wrongly described as a heart attack, although this can lead to a cardiac arrest they are two different conditions. A heart attack is a blockage, or partial blockage in one of the arteries that supplies blood to the heart, leading to tissue death. A cardiac arrest on the other hand is where the electrical signals to the heart are scrambled leading to ventricular fibrillation, which is where the heart becomes a like a quivering jelly. When the heart is randomly quivering like this it no longer pumps blood round the body effectively. Therefore, in basic terms, a heart attack is a plumbing issue and cardiac arrest is an electrical issue.

We deal with this electrical issue in much the same way as we deal with a computer that has crashed and frozen; we switch it off and back on again in the hope that when it restarts it will be functioning normally. That is what the defibrillator does, it sends and electrical current across the heart, effectively switching it off in an attempt to reset it.

There are two heart rhythms that can potentially be rectified with a shock from a defibrillator; they are ventricular fibrillation (VF) that we have just discussed, and ventricular tachycardia (VT) in which the heart is beating so fast that is no longer works effectively.

Implantable Cardioverter Defibrillator

An implantable cardioverter defibrillator (ICD) is a small device that can be surgically implanted beneath a person's skin and is designed to deliver a shock in much the same way as an AED does, manage the heart rate as a pacemaker does, or carry out cardioversion. Cardioversion is basically a series of shocks that restore the normal rhythm of the heart.

These are often fitted in patients who have a condition that can cause sudden cardiac arrest or abnormal heart rhythms. ICD's are fitted just underneath the collarbone, normally on the right side of the chest.

It is important to remember that if your patient has an ICD and they are in cardiac arrest, then it has probably stopped working, or is not working properly.

Using an Automated External Defibrillator

When training members of the public to carry out CPR and use a defibrillator, the thing that people are most afraid of is the defibrillator.

The biggest benefit of the AED is that they can be used by anyone, even those who have not had any training. The machine gives a running commentary from the moment the lid is opened, the electrodes come with diagrams that show the user where to place them, and the point that usually allays people's fears is the fact that an AED will not shock a heart that is beating normally.

Safety First

Firstly, some safety points to observe. There are certain places where operating an AED would be just too much of a risk. We all know that electricity and water do not mix and one of the more obvious hazards is standing water. Defibrillators can be used when it is raining, but if your patient is lying in a puddle of water, you should move them first.

Flammable atmospheres such as carbon monoxide from faulty domestic appliances or filling station forecourts are also a significant hazard, and before using a defibrillator your patient should be moved to a place of safety. Defibrillators are not classed as an intrinsically safe device, meaning that they may create a spark that could ignite flammable gases.

The final hazard to watch out for is metal surfaces such as fire escapes and mezzanine floors. Electrical current will take the path of least resistance, and if that happens to be through the patient and into the metal surface that you are kneeling on, then you are potentially risking a nasty shock yourself.

Prepare the Patient

Before attaching the electrodes there are a few things we need to look for first; I remember these as the five P's.

Pacemakers	Generally, these are found on the upper left hand side of the chest, if they are on the right hand side of the chest the electrode should be placed around 10 – 15cm away from the device.
Pendants	Remove any necklaces, or if this is not practical then the can be placed around the back of the patient.
Patches	Patches such as nicotine, or GTN (for angina) should be removed. Stick these on the side of your defibrillator or somewhere else as a reminder as to what patches the patient was using.
Perspiration	The patient may well be excessively sweaty, the chest should be dried quickly in the areas where the electrodes are to be connected using a cloth.
Piercings	If the patient has a piercing in their chest in the area where you need to attach an electrode, and it cannot be removed simply cover it entirely with the electrode. Time is important, and should not be wasted trying to remove a piercing.

Another consideration when preparing the patient is excessive chest hair. The defibrillator should come with a bag containing a safety razor, which can be used to remove any excessive chest hair in the areas where the electrodes will be placed. Again, this should be a quick process.

Electrode Placement

Most if not all AED's on the market come with diagrams on the electrode packaging, these show the user where to position the electrodes. The principle is that when the electrodes are placed correctly, the electrical current will follow the natural path that the body's electrical current follows as it travels across the heart, from the right shoulder across the heart to just beneath the left axilla or armpit.

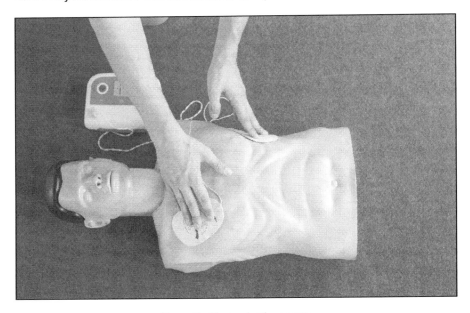

Figure 9 - Electrode Placement

Delivering a Shock

The AED will analyse the patient's heart rhythm at regular intervals and will announce this audibly. The device will ask everyone to stand clear of the patient; you also need to stay still as excessive movement can void the analysis and the device will have to repeat the process.

Following the analysis, the device will either tell the user to commence CPR or will advise a shock. At this point, the button will flash indicating that the device is ready to deliver a shock; supplementary oxygen **MUST** be removed prior to delivering a shock. Following the delivery of a shock the device will analyse again and either recommend another shock or ask the user to continue CPR.

Prior to delivering a shock, the user **MUST** ensure that nobody is touching the patient, and before pressing the button you should check the patient from head to toe to ensure that nobody is in contact.

Return of Spontaneous Circulation

More commonly referred to as ROSC, return of spontaneous circulation occurs following defibrillation when the heart restarts in normal sinus rhythm following a shock, this leads to the return of blood circulation around the body.

When this occurs the patient should be placed in the recovery position with the defibrillator electrodes left in place, if they are removed they are unlikely to stick to the body effectively if they are re-applied later. There is a chance your patient may go back into cardiac arrest so you should be prepared to roll them back over and start CPR.

Recovery Position

If our patient's ABC's are ok but they are unconscious, or they recover following defibrillation then they should be placed in what is known as the recovery position. The recovery position helps to maintain the patient's airway and prevents them from choking if they vomit.

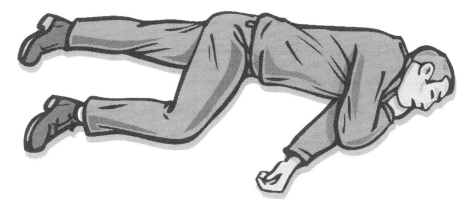

Figure 10 - Recovery Position

To place someone in the recovery position follow these simple steps:

- Kneel down next to your patient;
- Take the arm nearest to you and place it at a right angle to their body;
- Take the other hand and place the back of it against the cheek nearest to you and hold it in place;
- With your other arm lift up the knee furthest away from you as far as you can;
- Using the raised leg as a lever, roll the patient over towards you so that their head is resting on their arm and their cheek is still on their hand, and
- Tilt their head back to open the airway and raise their knee as shown in figure 5.

Once your patient has been placed in the recovery position you can carry out a secondary assessment known as the secondary survey and continue to monitor their ABC's. If the patient has been shocked by a defibrillator, circulation has returned and they are now breathing, you should leave the defibrillator electrodes on just in case they go back into cardiac arrest.

You should place a pregnant woman on their right side where possible. This is because the inferior vena cava, which is the main route for blood returning to the heart from the lower body, runs up the left hand side of the abdominal cavity and can be squashed by the baby, reducing the volume of blood flowing back to the heart.

Trauma

With emergencies involving physical trauma the theory that 'simple skills save lives' is as relevant as it is in medical emergencies. As a CFR we cannot crack open someone's chest, or intubate a patient, but what we can do is attempt maintain their basic life functions until someone who can arrives. A person stands a far greater chance of survival when someone arrives on scene quickly, controls bleeding, administers oxygen and, if necessary carries out CPR. It is the simple skills that keep the patient alive long enough for the paramedics and doctors to do what they do. Take that early intervention out of the equation and the patient's chances of survival fall dramatically.

Mechanism of Injury

A term you will come across regularly in the field of trauma is mechanism of injury. Mechanism of injury basically means how the injury occurred. An example of this would be:

"The head injury occurred as a result of the patient falling backwards from a 3 step ladder and striking the back of their head on a tiled kitchen floor"

Falls

Elderly people with mobility issues are particularly vulnerable to falls; this can be a very stressful and traumatic event, particularly where the individual involved lives alone. It is important to remember though, that anyone can be involved in a fall, no matter how old they are.

Management

The management of falls can range from simply helping someone up, to those involving fractures or head injuries. Sometimes it is the case that an elderly person has fallen from their own height and cannot get up on their own; they may need helping back into a chair and reassuring. In cases that are more serious the patient may have fallen from a height, such as down a set of stairs.

As a solo responder, it may not be possible to help somebody up safely on your own, and you may risk injury by trying to lift outside of your capabilities leaving the ambulance crew with two people to help. It is important to remember when lifting that you must be aware of your own capabilities and must never put yourself or the patient at risk.

Firstly, if your patient is alert and responsive you can ask them what happened. If they are not you should look for visual clues as to the distance somebody has fallen; if they are at the bottom of a set of stairs then potentially they have fallen from the top; there may be a ladder in the room, or they may be lying at the side of the bed.

If they are unconscious there is a reasonable chance that either they have fallen from a height and hit their head, suffered a head injury during a fall from their own height, or something medical caused the fall. Putting this together with visual clues such as fallen ladders can help you to put a picture together of what happened.

Unconscious Patient

Firstly, never forget to check for danger; after all, we do not yet know why our patient is unconscious on the floor!

For trauma incidents we add an extra 'C' to DR C ABCDE, it is just a little one and it comes after the A. Where we suspect that the patient may have injured their c-spine, we will consider it when managing their airway. To cover this we have DR C A(c)BCDE.

Instead of a head tilt chin lift, a jaw thrust should be carried out on a patient with a suspected c-spine injury; this is to avoid unnecessary movement of the neck.

Carry out a primary survey checking their airway, breathing and circulation. When checking their airway it is important to consider the potential for c-spine injuries, especially when a person has fallen from height. Where a c-spine injury is suspected you should maintain their airway without placing them in the recovery position, as doing so may cause further injury.

Check for visual signs of a head injury, and if it falls within your scope of practice, you can check the patient's pupils with a pen torch to see if they are equal in size and reactive to light.

Carry out a full secondary survey, record their breathing rate, pulse, blood pressure, and check their SPO^2. Supplementary oxygen can be given to maintain normal levels but does not need to be given routinely.

Do not forget to update your control room with further details.

> **Note:**
> Never forget to keep your patient warm, especially when outdoors. Cold patients do not tend to do as well as warm ones!

The Conscious Patient

The conscious patient may be more straight forward in terms of information gathering; I say may be easier because there is no guarantee that they will remember the events leading up to them being on the floor.

Firstly, speak to your patient, reassure them and try to find out what happened. If they have been on the floor for a significant length of time, as is sometimes the case, you should consider that they may be cold and frightened. If you cannot move them into a chair or back into bed then you need to make them as comfortable as possible and ensure that they are warm.

Next, take their medical history and a full set of observations including blood pressure, blood glucose, breathing rate, pulse rate and SPO^2. Try to build a picture of what happened; did a medical condition cause them to fall or did they simply trip over something and could not get back up? Use visual clues alongside the patient observations and medical history.

A full secondary survey should be carried out to check for injuries caused by the fall, ask the patient if they think that they could stand up with some assistance. If you suspect that they have an injury such as a fracture that could be made worse by attempting to stand then it may be better to leave them in a comfortable position until further help arrives.

Head Injuries

Head injuries can range from a mild concussion to a severe injury involving a bleed on the brain. The brain, for obvious reasons is quite important, it analyses information from our sensors and controls our vital systems such as breathing, which I think you will agree is pretty important. The brain is protected by our skull, three layers of protective tissue called dura mater, arachnoid mater and pia mater, and fluid called cerebrospinal fluid.

Different areas of the brain control different functions; they are the frontal lobe, parietal lobe, temporal lobe, occipital lobe, cerebellum and the brain stem. Brain injuries, depending on where they occur can therefore affect different functions.

When somebody is hit on the head or falls and hits their head on something with enough force they can be knocked out. There are different theories on why this occurs, one of which is that the impact imparts enough energy into the brain to affect the electrical signals, a bit like the reset that occurs when we shock the heart, or what happens when someone has a seizure. Now, plenty of people claim to have been knocked out, some clues as to whether they have or not include whether they can remember the events leading up to the injury and how they are immediately after regaining consciousness. Someone who has been knocked out will be somewhat confused and a little groggy when they come round, much like someone who is post ictal following a seizure; if they can remember events leading up to the injury and they are fully alert following, then the chances are that they were not knocked out.

Management

With a significant head injury, we should also be considering c-spine injuries, as a heavy blow to the head is likely to involve some force through the neck. When managing the airway of a patient with a suspected c-spine injury, a jaw thrust rather than head tilt chin lift should be carried out. You should also avoid placing your patient in the recovery position where a c-spine injury is suspected.

Assess the patient's level of consciousness using the AVPU scale (response) and then check their ABC's. If your patient is unconscious and not breathing then commence CPR.

Where your patient is unconscious and breathing check their pupils to see if they are equal and react to light, one pupil significantly larger than the other or pupils that do not react to light are a sign that a significant head injury has occurred. Where you suspect a serious head injury you should update your control room as this may require an upgraded response.

A conscious patient who was unconscious for any period because of a head injury will be confused when they regain consciousness, it is important to reassure your patient, but be aware that they may become combative due to the injury.

Supplementary oxygen should not be given routinely for head injuries and should be based on an assessment of the patient's SPO^2.

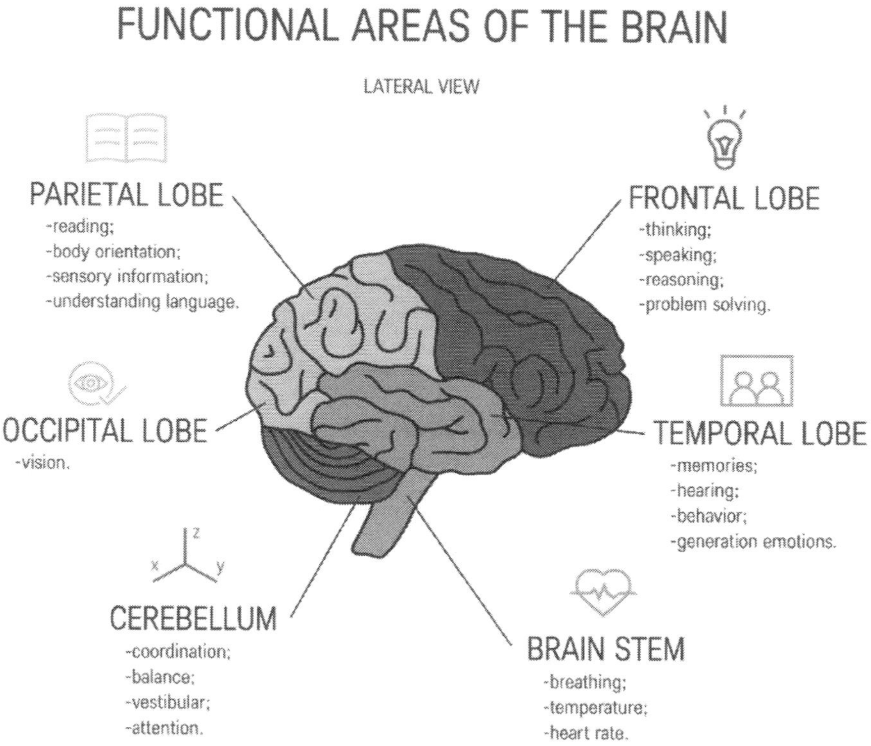

FUNCTIONAL AREAS OF THE BRAIN

LATERAL VIEW

PARIETAL LOBE
-reading;
-body orientation;
-sensory information;
-understanding language.

FRONTAL LOBE
-thinking;
-speaking;
-reasoning;
-problem solving.

OCCIPITAL LOBE
-vision.

TEMPORAL LOBE
-memories;
-hearing;
-behavior;
-generation emotions.

CEREBELLUM
-coordination;
-balance;
-vestibular;
-attention.

BRAIN STEM
-breathing;
-temperature;
-heart rate.

Figure 11 - Functional Areas of the Brain

Eye Injuries

Eye injuries can be very traumatic for the patient particularly where an object is lodged in the eye. The eyes are a key sensory organ allowing us to see the world around us. Anything that affects this vision can be very distressing.

Eye injuries may also occur because of blunt trauma, chemical splashes, burns, and dust or grit in the eye.

Management

As with any other penetrating injury involving an embedded object it is important not to remove the object or put pressure on it with a dressing. In order to cover the injured eye you will first need to place something over the penetrating object; plastic eye baths or similar are very useful for this purpose.

It is also important to cover the uninjured eye as well; this reduces movement of the injured eye. Try moving one eye independently from the other, it is almost impossible to do, and even if you can, it requires a lot of concentration. Covering the patients uninjured eye will help to reduce movement in both the uninjured eye and the injured eye.

Where there is dust or other foreign objects causing irritation the eye can be irrigated using eyewash. Where the irritation is as a result of a chemical the affected eye should be irrigated with copious amounts of irrigation fluid, saline solution or water for 20 to 30 minutes (NICE, 2017)

Eye injuries resulting from burns should be treated the same as a burn and then the eyes should be covered following a period of cooling with water. If there are burns to the eyes then the chances are there may be burns to airway and this will be your initial priority.

Human Eye Anatomy

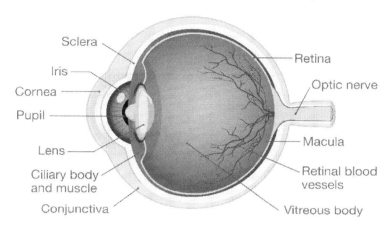

Figure 12 - The Human Eye

Ciliary Body and Muscle	Contraction of the ciliary muscle alters the shape of the lens allowing focus.
Conjunctiva	The mucous membrane that covers the front of the eye and the inside of the eyelids.
Cornea	The cornea is the transparent circular part at the front of the eye, which refracts light onto the lens.
Iris	Regulates the amount of light entering the eye.
Lens	Focuses the light entering the eye onto the retina
Optic Nerve	Passes visual information to the brain.
Pupil	Opening in the centre of the eye, which dilates and contracts allowing light into the lens.
Retina	Light sensitive layer that lines the inside of the eye.
Sclera	The white outer layer of the eyeball.
Vitreous Body	Clear jelly like material that fills the eyeball.

Table 7 - Key Components of the Human Eye

Bleeding

Blood is important stuff, it transports oxygen and nutrients around the body, and carries waste products to the relevant organs for disposal; blood also carries hormones, which are chemical messengers that tell the body's cells how to act, and electrolytes that control muscle contraction, manage the blood's PH level and transmit nerve impulses.

Blood consists of plasma, a straw-coloured fluid, which has different types of blood cells suspended in it.

Blood Cells	
Red Blood Cells (Erythrocytes)	99% of all blood cells are red blood cells. Their main function is to transport gases, mostly oxygen but some carbon dioxide.
Platelets (Thrombocytes)	Platelets contain a variety of substances that help with blood clotting, which causes bleeding to stop (Haemostasis).
White Blood Cells (Leukocytes)	White blood cells are engaged in defence and immunity; they detect foreign and abnormal materials and employ a number of mechanisms in order to destroy them.

Table 8 - Blood Cells

The body simply cannot function without blood, making the control of major bleeding essential.

Types of Bleed

There are three types of bleed, which are arterial, venous and capillary. The blood is carried around our body by arteries, veins and capillaries. The arteries carry oxygenated blood from the heart under pressure; because of this pressure, you get the characteristic spurting flow. This blood will generally be bright red in colour because of its higher oxygen content.

Venous pressure is lower and as a result you get a characteristic slow ooze. This blood tends to be darker in colour because of the reduced oxygen content. It is generally thought that a venous bleed is not as serious as an arterial bleed, but as they can be less obvious and easier to miss, an untreated venous bleed can be life threatening as well, particularly in patients who take anticoagulants or suffer from a clotting disorder.

Capillary bleeds are associated with scrapes and grazes and the blood flow is generally described as a trickle, these are not normally life threatening, although large scrapes and grazes have the potential to be a source of infection if they are not cleaned and covered.

Management

When looking for bleeding there is a method known as 'blood on the floor and four more'. This refers to obvious external bleeding (on the floor) and the major areas where internal bleeding can occur; the chest cavity (thorax), the abdomen, the pelvic cavity and the long bones for example the femur.

Small bleeds should be relatively easy to deal with using basic kit such as ambulance dressings and a little bit of well-directed pressure; major bleeds involving arteries can be more difficult.

Depending on your kit and level of training, you may be able to apply a purpose made trauma dressing. The Olaes Modular Bandage is particularly good as it has hook and loop (Velcro) strips along its length so that when it is applied tightly it does not slacken off if you drop it, it also has a plastic cup on the dressing to assist with the application of direct pressure to the source of the bleed.

If subsequent dressings have failed to control the bleed, the final option is a tourniquet. The application of a tourniquet should be seen as a last resort but can be very effective at controlling an arterial bleed if properly applied. The key to applying a tourniquet is pulling the strap as tight as possible before using the windlass; if the strap is tight enough then the windlass should only require 2 to 3 turns to control the bleed. If the first fails to control the bleed then a second can be applied.

Once a tourniquet has been applied, it should be left in place. Previously it was recommended that the tourniquet be released periodically to ensure that some blood flow is maintained to the limb; this is no longer recommended as the sudden release of blood can affect any clotting that has occurred, and if this is done frequently, the patient may potentially lose a significant amount of blood. Put it on and leave it on.

Tourniquet Application

The Royal College of Surgeons of Edinburgh – Faculty of Pre-Hospital Care recommends the following:

- Tourniquets should be considered a last resort, used when other methods have failed;
- In traumatic amputations a tourniquet should always be used;
- The tourniquet is applied as close to the wound as possible;
- Where the first is ineffective a second tourniquet should be applied above the first;
- Should be applied directly to skin, and
- Applied tightly enough to stop the bleed.

(FPHC, 2017)

Remember: Always act within your scope of practice and follow all trust policies and procedures.

Shock

> **DEFINITION**
> "**Shock is a life threatening generalised form of acute circulatory failure associated with inadequate oxygen utilisation by the cells**" (Cecconi, et al., 2014).

Shock is basically the failure of the circulatory system to adequately deliver oxygenised blood to the body's cells meaning that they fail to function properly. Shock can be broken down into three basic types; a problem with the pump, a lack of fluid to pump or poor distribution of the fluid meaning that there is not enough for every function.

Shock is not a condition itself, it occurs as a result of an injury or illness, so in effect it is a symptom of something else. It can be life threating and as such it needs to be managed.

To use the overused analogy of the central heating system, the system fails if the pump fails, and will not work effectively if the pump is failing. Another issue faced is low water pressure; if the volume of water in the system falls below a certain level then the heating system shuts down. In shock, the pump relates to the heart, and the water is the blood.

Low blood volume, which can occur as a result of internal or external bleeding, severe burns or dehydration is known as hypovolemic shock, the pump issue which can occur because of a heart attack for example, is known as cardiogenic shock.

For the third category, think about what happens if you turn on all the taps in your house at the same time, they will all start to lose pressure, some may even stop running altogether. This is because there is simply not enough capacity in the system to run all the taps at once, after all, this is not something you would normally do. With this type of shock all the blood vessels in the body dilate, increasing their capacity, meaning that there is not enough blood to fill them all. This is usually down to a severe infection such as sepsis.

Signs and symptoms that may indicate shock include:

- Mechanism of injury indicating internal bleeding.
- Severe infection such as sepsis;
- Severe burns;
- Pale clammy skin;
- Rapid weak pulse;
- Slow capillary refill time (greater than 2 seconds), and
- Confusion or anxiety.

Management of Shock

If you suspect shock then your patient needs immediate medical assistance. You should administer supplementary oxygen at 15 litres per minute and update your control room with your suspicions. If you have access to a clinical support hub then it may be worth calling for additional advice and triage.

Manage any external bleeding immediately and monitor for signs of internal bleeding. Shock itself is a sign of internal bleeding. You should also take into account any mechanism of injury such as suspected blunt force injury and other signs and symptoms.

Reassure your patient and carry out regular observations including respiratory rate, pulse rate, temperature and blood pressure and have these ready to hand over to the ambulance crew when they arrive. You can also check your patient's perfusion by carrying out a capillary refill test, normally the blood should return in under 2 seconds.

Try and keep your patient warm using blankets, particularly where they are outdoors.

Spinal Injuries

Injuries involving the spine are always a worry; the spine carries the spinal cord, and damage to the spinal cord can lead to partial or full paralysis and even death depending on where the cord is damaged. Thankfully, unstable spinal injuries are rare, and it requires a lot of force to fracture the spine.

Injuries involving the cervical spine or c-spine are always the most worrying as the nerves that control breathing run through this part of the spinal column, as well as the nerves that control movement in the upper and lower body.

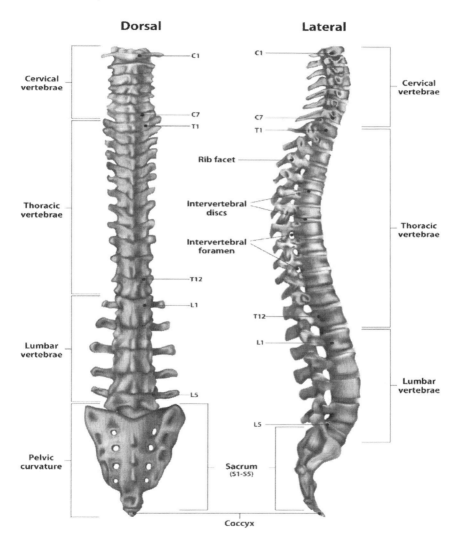

Figure 13 - Spinal Column

Management

Where spinal injury is suspected your first action should be to ensure that your patient remains immobile, preferably on their back lying straight with their head in line with their back and their legs straight.

If your patient is outside remember to keep them warm.

Ascertain through questioning of the patient or witnesses to see if there is any mechanism of injury suggestive of a spinal injury.

Check for any loss of sensation, pins and needles or tingling in the extremities.

Ask the patient whether they have suffered any previous spinal injuries or had any surgery on their spine.

Take a set of observations including blood pressure, respiratory rate, pulse rate and SPO^2.

Do not forget to check for other injuries.

> Note:
> Where any spinal fracture is suspected, do not attempt to move your patient unless their life is in immediate danger from an external factor such as fire.

Fractures

Fractures can range from minor, to life-threatening emergencies depending on their severity and location. Minor fractures rarely constitute a life-threatening situation, and in the majority of cases, someone with a minor fracture can make their own way to the nearest accident and emergency department or urgent care centre. Long bone fractures (femur for example), pelvic fractures, skull fractures and some open fractures can become life threatening emergencies due to the potential for severe blood loss, or in the case of skull fractures swelling or bleeding affecting the brain, which may in turn affect the function of vital organs within the body.

Fractures may occur due to direct force i.e. force applied directly to the fractured bone itself. They can occur because of indirect force, where the force is transferred through other bones until it reaches a relatively weak point causing a fracture, an example of this would be a frontal impact in a vehicle in which force is transferred through the lower limbs into the pelvis causing a pelvic fracture. Fractures can also occur for pathological reasons, such as disease.

Pelvic fractures are particularly troublesome as the aorta splits into the right and left common iliac (supplying blood to the legs) and internal iliac arteries; the corresponding veins also run through the pelvic cavity. Combine these vessels with sharp bone fragments and a cavity large enough to take most of the body's blood volume and you can see why a pelvic fracture can quickly become a life threatening condition.

Potential Blood Loss from Fractures	
Fracture	**Potential Loss (Litres)**
Ankle with moderate to severe swelling	0.25 to 0.5
Femur with moderate swelling	0.5 to 1
Femur with severe swelling	up to 4
Lower leg with moderate swelling	0.5 to 1
Forearm with moderate swelling	0.5 to 1
Pelvis	up to 5
Figures should be doubled for open fractures	

Table 9 - Blood Loss from Fractures

Signs and Symptoms

Fractures will need to be diagnosed by an x-ray; there are however some signs and symptoms that can lead you to suspect the one has occurred:

Limbs	Pelvis
Pain	as limbs plus:
Swelling	Shortening of one leg
Unnatural movement	Feet lying in abnormal/unequal positions
Crepitus (Grating Noise)	Mechanism of injury indicating possible pelvic fracture
Difficulty moving	
Mechanism of injury indicates a potential fracture	
Loss of strength in the affected limb, or Shock	
A diagnosed illness leading to bone weakness	

Management

Where available, Entonox may be administered for fractures unless contra-indicated (see chapter on pharmacology).

Immobilise the fracture site using a splint where available.

Take a set of observations, particularly where the reason for the injury is unclear i.e. did a medical episode lead to a fall?

Ascertain the mechanism of injury; a fall may have resulted in other injuries that are being masked due to the pain form the fracture.

Additional Action for Open Fractures

Manage any external haemorrhage.

If further advice is required, contact your trust's trauma cell.

You should not attempt to move of straighten the injured limb unless it falls within your scope of practice.

Dislocations

Dislocation is the separation of a joint. As with fractures, they can occur because of direct force, indirect force, or for pathological reasons. Dislocations can be extremely painful. Dislocations have the potential to cause nerve damage and affect the blood flow in the affected limb.

Signs and symptoms of a dislocation include significant deformation, reduced movement in the joint, pain and a mechanism of injury indicative of a dislocation.

Management

Do not attempt to relocate the joint.

Patients will tend to place the injured limb in a position that causes them the least pain, and you should not attempt to move it in any way.

Where you can, assist in supporting the limb using cushions or rolled up blankets.

Administer Entonox where available and not contra-indicated.

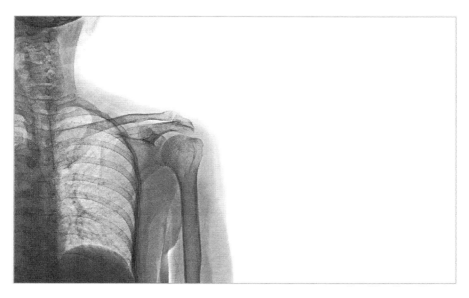

Figure 14 - Shoulder Dislocation

Chest Injuries

The chest cavity contains three of the most vital organs in the body; the heart and lungs. Damage to the lungs can reduce the amount of oxygen we can acquire from the atmosphere and damage to the heart can prevent that oxygen from being delivered to the vital organs.

A damaged lung, from a broken rib for example, can cause air to enter the chest cavity causing a serious condition known as a pneumothorax (***pneumo relating to air and thorax relating to the chest cavity***). Where the damage affects blood vessels or the heart the chest cavity can fill with blood, this is known as a haemothorax (***haemo relating to blood***). Both of these conditions can cause a lung to collapse vastly reducing the amount of oxygen that the body can acquire from the atmosphere.

When one or more ribs break in two places there will be a section of free floating ribs, this is known as flail chest.

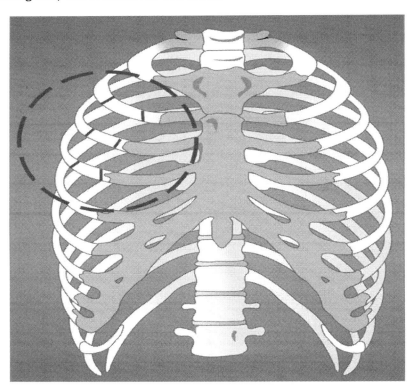

Figure 15 - Flail Chest Segment

Management

If an object such as a piece of glass is still embedded in the wound you should not try to remove it as this may potentially cause further damage and increase internal bleeding. A dressing should be rolled up in a donut shape and placed around the object, a bandage can then be placed over this to hold it in place; it is important that the bandage is not placed over the object and is simply applied either side of it.

Internal Injuries

Internal bleeding may not be obvious at first as the human body has a capacity to compensate for blood loss up to a certain level, after this, your patient can suddenly and rapidly deteriorate.

Signs that could lead you to suspect internal bleeding include:

- Known or suspected blunt force injury;
- Heavy bruising;
- Pallor of the skin;
- Sweating;
- Rapid weak pulse, and
- Increased respiratory rate.

Management

Unfortunately as a first responder we are limited in what we can do for a patient with internal injuries, what the patient needs is a surgeon. Managing the patient with internal bleeding as a CFR involves monitoring their ABC's, SpO^2 levels, pulse, capillary refill, and blood pressure, and providing reassurance; it is also important to update the control room when internal bleeding is suspected.

Burns

Burns can range in size and severity, from minor scalds to deep full thickness burns affecting large areas of the body. The area of the body affected can also affect the severity; for example, a scald on the arm would be seen as relatively minor compared to burns affecting the airway, or those that stretch all the way around the chest.

Superficial	Involving only the outer most layer of the skin, superficial burns appear red and when pressed will blanch and then return to a red colour. Blisters do not usually occur with this type of burn.
Partial Thickness	Partial thickness burns involve the epidermis and dermis. The skin will be red in colour and will blanch when touched, turning white and then red again. Blisters will be present with partial thickness burns.
Full Thickness	Full thickness burns involve the destruction of both the epidermis and dermis. The skin will be pale and waxy or charred. The patient may not feel any pain due to the destruction of the sensory nerves. The areas around the full thickness burns will still probably be painful and will consist of areas of partial thickness and superficial burns.

Management

The rule of nines is a method of estimating the area of burns on your patient's body. Each part of the body represents a certain percentage of the total (see table 8).

Rule of Nines	
Front and back of head	9%
Front and back of arms	9% per arm
Front and back of legs	18% per leg
Anterior trunk (front)	18%
Posterior trunk (back)	18%
Groin	1%

Table 10 - Rule of Nines

There is also a handy app available on the App Store that allows the user to select the burn depth and colour in the affected area on an outline body; the app then calculates the estimated area. To download you can scan the QR code in table 9.

Mersey Burns app for iPhone
A free app for calculating burn area percentages

Table 11 - Mersey Burns App

Cut away any smouldering clothing but do not remove anything that is stuck to the skin, and where possible remove any rings or jewellery that may affect circulation when swelling occurs.

Cool the burn using cool water continuously for around 20 minutes. The water should be cool but not freezing cold as this can make things worse. Do not interrupt cooling until the 20 minutes is up.

Burns present the risk of infection as the damaged tissue provides a route for bacteria to enter the body. Cover the burn with a suitable non-adherent dressing; cling film is particularly good for this. Never wrap the cling film around the affected area, any subsequent swelling will cause it to tighten potentially affecting circulation. Simply lay the cling film over the affected area.

Assess you patient for signs of shock due to fluid loss. A significant amount of fluid can be lost as a result of severe burns and shock is a significant risk factor in burns patients.

For burns affecting the airway, it is important that the airway is managed and maintained. Airway adjuncts such as oropharyngeal airways can be used if they are provided by your trust and you are trained to use them.

Circumferential burns, that is burns that stretch all the way around the body, for example all the way round the chest or neck, are very serious and can cause breathing or circulation issues. As the skin burns, it tightens, preventing the chest from expanding properly, or constricting the patient's airway. If this happens you should contact your control room as this is potentially life threatening.

> **Remember**
> **Cool the burn; warm the patient. Limit your cooling efforts to the area of the burn itself but try to keep your patient warm.**

Secondary Survey

Once the immediately life threatening stuff has been ruled out it is time to have a look for any other injuries. To do this we carry out a full head to toe assessment of our casualty, and it is important not to miss the areas that you would not normally want to look.

The secondary survey is a head to toe assessment of our patient looking for additional injuries such as bruising, bleeding and fractures. The injuries we worry about the most tend to be head injuries and injuries to the spinal column, followed by the chest, abdomen and pelvis, so it makes perfect sense to start with these, in that order. Once these have been checked you can then move onto the limbs.

Secondary Survey	
Head	Check all around the skull looking for: • Bruising; • Bleeding; • Lumps; • Straw coloured fluid or blood from the ears or nose. Check for bruising around both eyes as this can be an indicator of a skull fracture, and check whether both pupils are equal and react to light.
Neck	Again, you are looking for bruising and bleeding; you should check the cervical spine for signs of lumps, which may indicate a spinal injury. Look at the trachea (windpipe) if this has moved over to one side it may be an indication that there is a tension haemo or pneumothorax present.
Chest	Does the chest rise and fall equally on both sides, or is one part of the chest wall moving independently? Has anything penetrated the chest wall, or are there signs of blunt force trauma such as severe bruising?
Abdomen	Look for signs of blunt force trauma e.g. bruising and any penetrating wounds. Is there any tenderness when you touch the abdominal area?
Pelvis	Is there any bruising or bleeding? Are both feet lying equally, or is one lying in an abnormal position? Does one leg appear shorter than the other does?
Limbs	Check the limbs for abnormalities, bruising and bleeding.

Table 12 - Secondary Survey

Patient Questioning

Information gathering is a vital part of the decision making process and it is important that we gather all the relevant information in a timely manner in order to decide upon the best course of action for our patient. The way we ask the questions is also important, for example by asking closed questions, such as have you got pain in your chest, you may miss something important; instead, by asking have you got any pain anywhere you may get a completely different answer leading to a completely different diagnosis.

With closed questions, you also run the risk of confirmation bias, where the patient thinks they know what is wrong with them and they agree with what you are asking because they believe that it confirms their own diagnosis. A good method is to follow SAMPLE, which stands for signs and symptoms; allergies; medications; pertinent medical history; last oral intake (food or drink) and events leading up to the illness/accident.

S	Signs and symptoms: How does the patient look e.g. pale and clammy; are they breathing quickly or slowly; can they speak in full sentences or do the need to pause for breath between words?
A	Are they allergic to any medications?
M	What medication are they taking if any? (prescription or otherwise)
P	Pertinent medical history. Just the important stuff though, you don't need to know that your patient had measles in 1965, but it may be useful to know that they have recently been in hospital for heart surgery, or they have a family history of heart disease.
L	Last oral intake. When did they last have anything to eat or drink?
E	Events leading up to the illness/accident? Were they mowing the lawn, out jogging or snoozing on the sofa? This can be important and can help to distinguish between certain conditions, such as angina and a heart attack.

Table 13 - SAMPLE

Provided that you have asked all the relevant questions, don't beat yourself up if your patient gives a completely different version of events to the ambulance crew when they arrive. This happens from time to time, it is one of the job's little mysteries and I can guarantee it has happened to most responders at some point. I can still remember the first time a patient told me they were normally fit and well and then proceeded to reel off a list of medications for a variety of conditions when the crew arrived.

Health Conditions

As a community responder, you will be called to patients suffering from a range of health conditions, some of which will be pre-existing, some of which will be previously undiagnosed.

You will not be expected to have an encyclopaedic knowledge of all conditions, but a good understanding of some of the more common conditions is extremely beneficial.

Cardiac Conditions

The heart is a pump containing a series of valves that utilises muscle contractions to pump blood around the body. These muscle contractions are controlled by an electrical current that passes across the heart first contracting the atria and then the ventricles. In order to work efficiently then, the heart requires healthy muscle tissue, co-ordinated electrical signals from the brain and of course blood.

The blood follows a certain path through the heart to the lungs, and then back to the heart for distribution throughout the body. Used (or deoxygenated) blood is returned to the heart by the superior vena cava where it enters the right atrium, as the right atrium contracts the blood is squeezed into the right ventricle through a one-way valve called the tricuspid valve. From the right ventricle, the blood is then pumped out of the heart through the pulmonary artery to the lungs. On arrival in the lungs the blood gets rid of carbon dioxide and exchanges it for oxygen before heading back to the heart. The blood arrives back at the heart via the pulmonary vein into the left atrium, and from there it heads through another one-way valve called the Mitral Valve and from there it heads off around the body via the aorta.

Just like a car there are various components in the heart that can become faulty, or wear out, such as the valves or the muscle itself, and the arteries that supply blood to the heart can become partially or fully blocked.

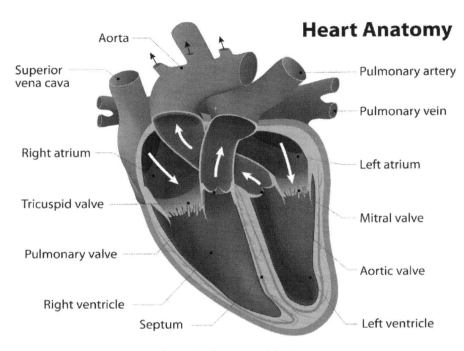

Figure 16 - Anatomy of the Heart

What we should not forget, is that as well as pumping blood to other organs around the body, the heart itself also needs oxygenated blood in order to survive.

Now we have discussed the plumbing, it would be prudent to work through the electrical system.

Muscles in the body contract because of electrical impulses, and the heart is no different. The electrical system in the heart consists of the Sinoatrial (SA) Node, the Atrioventricular (AV) Node, the bundle of His, the left bundle branch, left anterior division, right anterior division and the right bundle branch. Attached to these bundle branches are Purkinje Fibres.

The electrical current starts out at the SA node, which is the heart's built in pace maker and controls your heart rate based on the needs of the body. The impulses from the SA node pass through the atria causing them to contract, and then arrives at the AV node. At the AV node the impulse pauses briefly to allow all the blood to be pumped from the Atria to the ventricles.

Once the atria are empty the one-way valves close and the atria begin to refill with blood, the electrical impulses can now continue their journey to the bundle of his and then along the left and right bundle branches into the Purkinje fibres where they cause the ventricles to contract.

Heart Attack

A heart attack, also known as a myocardial infarction (MI) is caused by a blockage in the artery that supplies blood to the heart muscle. Without oxygenated blood the heart muscle will not function properly, and the tissue will start to die; the more of the heart muscle that dies the lower the patient's chance of survival.

Signs and Symptoms

Some symptoms of a heart attack include:

- Centralised crushing chest pain;
- Pain that spreads to other parts of the body such as the arms and jaw;
- Feeling light headed or dizzy;
- Coughing and/or wheezing;
- Nausea, and/or
- Overwhelming anxiety.

Not every patient will display all of these symptoms, and some patient may initially have very few symptoms at all.

Management

The first thing you should do if you suspect that your patient is having a heart attack is update your control room. If the initial information was not suggestive of this it is important that this information is passed back as the ambulance response can be re-prioritised.

You should sit the patient in a comfortable position, preferably on the floor with their back supported and their knees up; this is commonly known as the 'W' position. You should loosen any tight clothing and keep your patient as comfortable as possible while reassuring them.

If it is within your scope of practice and there is nothing to suggest that the patient is allergic, you can give a single 300mg dose of aspirin (1 tablet).

Supplementary oxygen should be given if your patients saturated oxygen levels fall below their normal rates of 94% to 98% for a non-COPD patient or 88% to 92% for a patient with COPD.

If your patient loses consciousness you should carry out a primary survey and be prepared to carry out CPR. If your patient does go into cardiac arrest it is very important that you update the control room again.

Angina

Angina is caused by a narrowing of the arteries that supply blood to the heart. The reduced blood flow to the heart means than on exertion the heart muscle cannot get enough oxygenated blood. Because of this, the chest pain relating to angina generally comes on following some kind of exercise or exertion.

Angina may be stable or unstable. Stable angina, which is not normally a life threatening condition, is the more common type. Stable angina, attacks normally have a trigger such as exercise and symptoms will usually pass within a few minutes of resting. Unstable angina is more serious and attacks can occur without a trigger; symptoms may also remain despite resting.

People who are diagnosed with angina will generally be prescribed Glyceryl Trinitrate (GTN), which can come in spray form, tablet form or in some cases as a patch. GTN causes blood vessels to dilate, taking the pressure of the heart and increasing blood flow.

Signs and Symptoms

Like a heart attack, one of the main symptoms of angina is chest pain, which may spread to other areas of the body. The pain may be described as a dull pain and the chest may feel tight and heavy. Some patients, especially women may suffer from a sharp stabbing pain. In angina, the pain comes on during exertion for example walking up a hill.

Other symptoms include:

- Tiredness;
- Nausea;
- Breathlessness, and/or
- Pain in the lower chest or stomach.

Management

As already discussed, your patient may already have their own GTN spray, and if they haven't taken it already they should be encouraged to. If this does not relieve their symptoms then this may be a sign of something more serious such as a heart attack.

You should monitor your patients breathing rate, pulse and SPO^2 and treat accordingly until the ambulance arrives and a 12 lead ECG can be done. If there is any significant deterioration in the patient's condition you should inform your control room immediately.

Heart Failure

More common in older people, heart failure basically means that the heart is no longer able to pump blood around the body effectively which normally occurs because the heart has become too weak or stiff. This does not mean that the heart has stopped working; it just needs some assistance to do its job properly.

Heart failure is a long-term condition for which there is generally no cure, treatment is usually based around controlling the symptoms.

Symptoms of heart failure include:

- Breathlessness.
- Swelling in the legs and ankles caused by fluid build-up.
- A persistent cough, which may be worse at night.
- Wheezing.
- Loss of appetite.
- Palpitations.
- Fast heart rate.
- Dizziness.

The most common causes of heart failure are a heart attack, high blood pressure and cardiomyopathy which is a disease of the heart muscle that can be either inherited or caused by viral infections (BHF, 2019)

Management

There is a good chance that your patient will be aware of their condition, they may have their own medication and will usually know if their condition is better or worse than normal.

As a CFR, you should ensure that the patient is comfortable, monitor their ABC's, SpO^2 levels, blood pressure, respiratory rate and pulse and administer supplementary Oxygen as required. It is important to record these observations and look for signs that their condition improving, getting worse or staying the same.

Stroke

A stroke occurs because of either a blockage in one of the vessels supplying blood to the brain (ischaemic stroke) or a bleed (haemorrhagic stroke). Both of these conditions cause an interruption in the blood flow to part of the brain, and given how important the brain is, and the fact that brain tissue dies without an adequate supply of oxygenated blood, a stroke is most definitely a serious life threatening condition.

Symptoms of a stroke include:

- FAST (Face, Arms, Speech, Tongue).
- One sided paralysis.
- Confusion.
- Dizziness.
- Balance and co-ordination problems.
- Problems understanding.
- Sudden and extremely severe headache.

Management

Carry out a primary survey.

Carry out a FAST test and if a stroke is indicated, you should update your control room.

F	A	S	T
Facial Weakness	**Arm Weakness**	**Speech**	**Tongue**
Has their face dropped on one side?	Can they hold both their arms out and hold them there?	Is their speech slurred?	Ask them to stick out their tongue; does it fall to one side?

Table 14 - FAST Test

Take your patient's blood pressure in both arms for comparison.

Monitor their SPO_2 levels and administer supplementary oxygen as required. Oxygen does not need to be administered routinely for a stroke and should only be given to maintain normal levels.

Reassure your patient and explain what is happening.

Continue monitoring their ABC's.

Respiratory Issues

The lungs work together with the heart to supply oxygen to the body; their job is to exchange carbon dioxide (a waste product) for oxygen. As discussed earlier, the lungs receive deoxygenated blood from the heart via the pulmonary artery, carbon dioxide is exchanged for oxygen and the oxygenated blood is returned to the heart via the pulmonary vein.

Atmospheric air is taken in (inspiration) via the nose and or mouth and into the naso/oropharynx, from there it passes through the epiglottis and into the larynx and trachea. The trachea splits into the left and right bronchi from where it enters the left and right lungs.

Once in the lungs the air passes through bronchioles eventually landing in the alveoli, this is where the gas exchange takes place.

Composition of Air				
	Oxygen (O^2)	Carbon Dioxide (CO^2)	Nitrogen (N)	Water Vapour
Inspired Air	21%	0.04%	78%	Variable
Expired Air	16%	4%	78%	Saturated

Table 15 - Composition of Air

Fact:
The pulmonary artery is the only artery in the body that carries deoxygenated blood, and the pulmonary vein is the only vein that carries oxygenated blood.

Used blood (deoxygenated) is carried to the lungs from the heart via the pulmonary artery, as it passes through the alveoli carbon dioxide is exchanged for oxygen and the blood is returned to the heart via the pulmonary vein. Approximately 5% of the inspired oxygen is used by the body, meaning that 16% remains; this is important when we carry out CPR.

Asthma

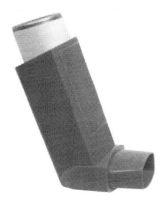

Figure 17 - Inhaler

The airway of an asthma sufferer is a bit like one of those irritable people, we have all met them, in fact on occasion I can be one of those people. They are easily irritated by certain things; for me it is people who talk on their phones when they are driving.

With asthma, the airways are irritable, and certain things can cause this to flare up. When an irritant is inhaled, such as pet dander, household dust or even cold air, the airways become inflamed and tighten this makes it more difficult to breathe and causes a feeling of tightness in the chest. The most noticeable sign that this has occurred is a wheezing sound, the patient may also be breathless, and they may be unable to speak in full sentences.

Common triggers include the common cold; Allergies to things such as pet hair or pollen; Irritants such as aerosol sprays or tobacco smoke; stress; Air pollution such as vehicle exhaust fumes and Running or exercising in cold weather (exercise-induced asthma).

Common symptoms of asthma include
- Shortness of breath;
- Wheezing on exhalation;
- Tightness in the chest, and
- Coughing.

Management

Reassure the patient and remove them from the trigger e.g. cold weather or dusty environment.

Encourage or assist the patient to use their own inhaler.

Monitor the patient's SPO^2 and administer supplementary oxygen as required.

Chronic Obstructive Pulmonary Disease

More commonly known as COPD, chronic obstructive pulmonary disease isn't a condition in itself, it is an umbrella term for a group of conditions that make it harder to expel all the air from the lungs.

People with COPD will generally have lower levels of saturated oxygen (SpO^2) in their blood.

Normal SpO2 Levels	94 to 98%
Normal SpO^2 Levels (COPD)	88 to 92%

Table 16 - Oxygen Levels

Management

A patient with COPD may have their own oxygen equipment, however if this is malfunctioning or their oxygen levels have dropped below their normal range they may require additional oxygen.

It may be better for your patient to use their existing mask or nasal cannula and simply connect it to your bottle.

Start at 2 litres per minute and increase by 2 litres per minute every 5 minutes, to a maximum of 10 litres until normal levels are reached.

If a nasal cannula is being used then it must be changed for a simple facemask when you exceed 6 litres per minute.

Choking

Choking can be extremely distressing for the patient whether it is a partial or full blockage, and a full blockage in particular can become a life threatening condition without early intervention. People who are choking will generally attempt to cough up the object, they will probably start to panic and some may even get up and leave the room to avoid making a scene.

Management

Firstly, you should encourage the patient to cough. This may or may not dislodge the item.

If coughing is unsuccessful or the patient is unable to cough, you should administer five back blows.

If the back blows are unsuccessful administer 5 chest thrusts and rotate between (see figure 17).

After each back blow or chest thrust check to see if the item has become dislodged; after all, you do not want to continue hitting your patient if it has!

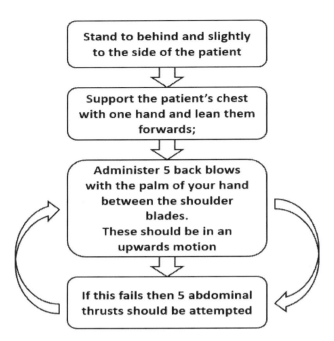

Figure 18 - Choking Flowchart

If you are unable to dislodge the item, be prepared for your patient to go into respiratory/cardiac arrest.

If the item is dislodged and expelled, carry out an assessment of your patient and take a set of observations.

Check their SPO^2 levels and administer supplementary oxygen as required.

Advise the patient to remain at the scene until the ambulance crew have been and checked them over.

Epilepsy

Epilepsy is a condition that affects the brain and causes frequent seizures (NHS, 2017). These seizures occur as a result of sudden bursts of electrical activity in the brain that temporarily affect how it functions. According to the charity Epilepsy Action, there are around 600,000 epilepsy sufferers in the UK making it one of the most common serious neurological conditions.

Management

Seeing someone have an epileptic fit for the first time can be a frightening experience and the key is to remain calm. As a first responder you cannot prevent or stop the fit, but you can prevent your patient from injuring themselves by moving any moveable furniture and placing a cushion under the patient's head. NEVER try and place anything, especially fingers, in the patient's mouth, as you are liable to receive a nasty bite as the muscles in the patient's jaw contract; there is also the risk of choking.

Once the fit is over the patient will be post-ictal, meaning that they will be confused and possibly quite frightened, they may also feel tired; fitting can be exhausting due to the constant muscle contractions, and may affect their SPO^2 levels. Where this is the case, you should administer supplementary oxygen as per your trust guidelines.

If this is the patient's first fit, or the fits are continuous with little or no break in between then the patient needs to go to hospital.

Diabetes

The primary organ involved here is the liver. The liver is responsible for carbohydrate metabolism and plays a vital role in maintaining blood glucose levels. In the liver, the hormone insulin stimulates the conversion of glucose into glycogen, which is then stored until required. When blood glucose levels fall another hormone, glucagon, steps up and stimulates the conversion of the stored glycogen back into glucose. When this process is running as it should, blood glucose levels are maintained within normal levels, however a condition known as diabetes can throw a spanner in the works.

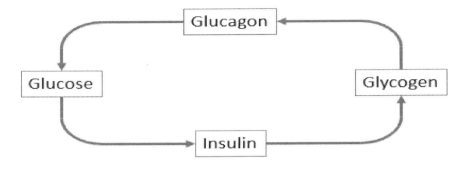

Figure 19 - Glucose Cycle

When your patient's blood sugar levels are high (see chart) they are classed as being hyperglycaemic (hyper = high) and when their levels are low they are classed as being hypoglycaemic (hypo = low).

Normal Blood Sugar Levels			
	Upon Waking	**Before Meals**	**At Least 90 minutes after meals**
Non-diabetic		4 to 5.9 mmol/L	Under 7.8 mmol/L
Type 1	5 to 7 mmol/L	4 to 7 mmol/L	5 to 9 mmol/L
Type 2		4 to 7 mmol/L	Under 8.5 mmol/L
Type 1 (Child)	4 to 7 mmol/L	4 to 7 mmol/L	5 to 9 mmol/L

Table 17 - Normal Blood Sugar Levels

There are 2 types of diabetes known as type 1 or type 2 which may be controlled by either medication or diet. Diabetes basically affects glucose levels in the blood and may cause levels to be dangerously high or low.

Type 1 diabetes, sometimes called insulin dependent diabetes is down to a severe deficiency or absence of insulin production and is more prevalent in children and young adults, in order to control type 1 diabetes is managed through insulin injections.

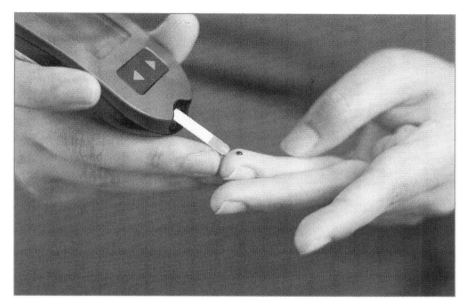

Figure 20 - Testing Blood Glucose Levels

Type 2 diabetes sometimes known as non-insulin dependent diabetes is the most common type of diabetes and around 90% of cases are type 2. In type 2 diabetes, changes can occur in the cell membranes preventing the glucose from entering the cells.

The onset of type 2 is slow, often over many years and can often go unnoticed.

Type 2 diabetes is treated with diet and/or drugs although in some cases injections may be required.

Management

Hypoglycaemia

Where available give Glucogel (40%) and follow with oral carbohydrates (a jam sandwich or similar is good for this), and

Reassess BM every 5 minutes (Target greater than 5.0).

<u>Hyperglycaemia</u>

If unconscious place in recovery position;

Monitor ABC's and O2 levels (consider supplementary O2 if levels drop);

Reassess BM every 5 minutes, and

Be prepared for the patient to go into cardiac arrest.

Sepsis

Sepsis is a serious life threatening condition that can cause the sufferers organs to shut down. The condition kills around 5 people per hour in the UK (Sepsis Trust, 2019), that's more people than breast, bowel and prostate cancer combined (Cox, 2017).

A basic description of Sepsis is that it is "the body's overreaction to an infection causing it to injure its own organs and tissues", so rather than being an infection, Sepsis is actually because of the body's response to an infection. It's a bit like getting a paper cut on your finger and instead of putting a plaster on it, you have the finger amputated.

Signs and Symptoms

The symptoms of sepsis can be very similar to influenza. The following signs and symptoms may indicate sepsis (NICE, 2017):

History

- Recent changes in behaviour and mental state;
- Recent loss of functional ability;
- Patient who is immunosuppressed, and
- Recent trauma or surgery.

Observations

- Respiratory rate greater than 25 breaths per minute;
- Systolic blood pressure between 91 and 100 mmHg;
- Heart rate greater than 130 beats per minute;
- Not passed urine in last 18 hours;

- Tympanic temperature less than 36°;
- Non-blanching rash (doesn't disappear under a glass), and
- Mottled ashen skin with cyanosis.

Table 18 uses the word sepsis as a method of remembering some of the potential indicators of sepsis.

S	Slurred Speech or Confusion
E	Extreme Shivering or Muscle Pain
P	Passing no Urine (In a Day)
S	Severe Breathlessness
I	It Feels Like you are Going to Die
S	Skin Mottled or Discoloured

Table 18 - SEPSIS indicators (Source: Sepsis Trust)

NEWS2

The national early warning score (NEWS), developed by the Royal College of Physicians, is a diagnosis tool that can be used to identify clinical deterioration in patients. The second version (NEWS2 was released in 2017 (NHS, 2017).

NEWS scores are based on a series of physiological parameters:

- Respiration rate;
- SpO^2 on air or oxygen;
- Systolic blood pressure;
- Pulse rate;
- Level of consciousness (ACVPU), and
- Temperature (°C).

Each of these physical parameters is scored depending on the results, for example a respiration rate of 22 would score a 2.

If this increased to 26 the score would rise to 3, indicating a possible clinical deterioration in the patient.

More information about NEWS2 can be found online, including a full colour copy of the NEWS2 scoring chart:

https://www.rcplondon.ac.uk/projects/outputs/national-early-warning-score-news-2

Physiological parameter	Score						
	3	2	1	0	1	2	3
Respiration rate (per minute)	≤8		9–11	12–20		21–24	≥25
SpO$_2$ Scale 1 (%)	≤91	92–93	94–95	≥96			
SpO$_2$ Scale 2 (%)	≤83	84–85	86–87	88–92 ≥93 on air	93–94 on oxygen	95–96 on oxygen	≥97 on oxygen
Air or oxygen?		Oxygen		Air			
Systolic blood pressure (mmHg)	≤90	91–100	101–110	111–219			≥220
Pulse (per minute)	≤40		41–50	51–90	91–110	111–130	≥131
Consciousness				Alert			CVPU
Temperature (°C)	≤35.0		35.1–36.0	36.1–38.0	38.1–39.0	≥39.1	

Figure 21 - NEWS2 (Source: Royal College of Physicians)

Management

Where sepsis is suspected, high flow oxygen should be administered via a non-rebreather/reservoir mask.

Take a patient history and assess the patient looking for sources of suspected infection.

Take a full set of observations and assess the patient against NEWS2 criteria or using your trust's sepsis screening tool.

Inform your control room and the attending paramedic/EMT that you suspect the patient may have sepsis.

Anaphylaxis

Anaphylaxis is the body's reaction to a substance (allergen) to which the sufferer is allergic to; common allergens include nuts, bee stings and shellfish. Anaphylaxis can be extremely serious and cause the patients airway to swell up leading to hypoxia.

Most known sufferers will carry an Epipen on their person, or will have one close to hand. An Epipen contains epinephrine, which is a chemical that narrows blood vessels and opens the airways in the lungs.

Anaphylaxis Criteria **Anaphylaxis is likely when the following criteria are met**
Sudden onset and rapid progression of symptoms
Life threatening airway and/or breathing and/or circulation problems
Skin changes such as urticaria (hives), flushing, angioedema (swelling of the skin)

Table 19 - Anaphylaxis Criteria

Cardiac or respiratory arrest may occur within minutes in severe cases and the upper airway may be compromised where the tongue is involved. Where the upper airway is involved, stridor may be noted. The patient may have a hoarse or quiet voice and may lose the ability to speak as the condition progresses. Audible chest wheezing is common.

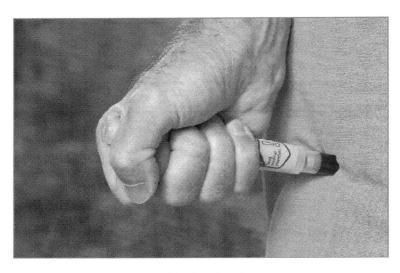

Figure 22 - Use of an Epipen

Management

Give supplementary oxygen at 15 litres/min via a non-rebreather mask, as per oxygen therapy guidelines.

Known sufferers may be carrying their own EpiPen (Epinephrine Autoinjector). Assist the patient to administer their own medication, or **IF SUITABLY TRAINED**, administer the epinephrine into the patient's thigh.

Monitor the patient's ABC's.

Hypothermia

Our body's core temperature is maintained within a very narrow range and should normally be between 36.5° and 37.5° Celsius; the problem is that our bodies are very good at losing heat, but not so great at generating it. When our body temperature reaches 35° or less we are classed as hypothermic.

Hypothermia can affect many functions of the body including the clotting process, meaning that hypothermic patients are particularly vulnerable when they have also suffered major trauma leading to haemorrhage, either internally or externally.

Signs and Symptoms

Mild (32°C - 35°C) – Uncontrolled shivering, patient still alert, mild confusion, lethargy, increased BP, pulse rate and respiratory rate may follow.

Moderate (30°C - 32°C) – Shivering slows or stops, mental confusion and apathy develop, slurred speech, BP drops, and breathing becomes slower.

Severe (<30°C) – Skin may be bluish-grey in colour, the patient is very weak, may appear drunk, gradual loss of consciousness.

Swiss staging model		
Stage	**Clinical findings**	**Core temp**
HT-I	Conscious, shivering	35°C to 32°C
HT-II	Impaired consciousness, not shivering	32°C to 28°C
HT-III	Unconscious, but vital signs present	28°C to 24°C
HT-IV	No vital signs	

Table 20 - Swiss Staging Model

Management

Where possible move the patient to a warmer environment.

Remove any wet clothing and replace with blankets and a foil blanket to help to keep any body heat in.

Do not give the patient any alcohol or hot drinks.

Administer high flow oxygen and monitor the patient's SPO_2.

The warming process should be gradual.

> **Note:**
> For extremes of body temperature a good rule of thumb to follow is 'warm slowly; cool quickly'.

Carbon Monoxide Poisoning

Carbon monoxide (CO) is produced by the incomplete combustion of carbon based fuels, such as gas, coal or wood; put basically, when these fuels burn and there is not enough oxygen to burn up all the fuel carbon monoxide is formed. Any household appliance that burns these fuels can produce carbon monoxide, for example, gas or oil fired boilers, gas fires, or wood burning stoves; the most common producers are faulty gas boilers or fires.

Carbon monoxide binds to the haemoglobin in the blood far easier than oxygen does, and as a result the oxygen in the blood is displaced and replaced with carbon dioxide creating carboxyhaemoglobin. A pulse oximeter sees carboxyhaemoglobin in the same way as it sees oxygenated blood, therefore a patient with carbon monoxide poising may present with perfectly normal SpO^2 levels.

As well as being fatal through inhalation, carbon monoxide gas is also flammable and accumulations within a confined space can form an explosive atmosphere.

I carry a cheap carbon monoxide detector with my kit, this may give an early warning of the presence of carbon monoxide. They can be purchased at most good DIY stores.

Signs and Symptoms (NICE, 2018)

Brief Exposure	
Low Levels	**High Levels**
Flushed skin	Confusion
Dizziness	Loss of consciousness; death
Headache	Movement problems
Nausea and vomiting	Heart attack
Aching muscles	Respiratory arrest
Confusion	Weakness

Longer Term Exposure to Low Levels	
Cardiovascular problems	
Dizziness	Flu like symptoms
Dementia	Tiredness
Headache	Lethargy
Loss of vision	Memory problems
Nausea	Loss of balance
Sleep issues	Altered sense of smell
Anxiety	Personality issues

Management

Do not put yourself at unnecessary risk.

If you can move the patient outdoors and away from the source then you should do so.

Open doors and windows if it safe to do so.

Isolate the gas supply at the meter if safe to do so. Normally if the valve lever is in line with the pipe then the gas is on; if it is at 90 degrees to the pipe then the gas is off.

Administer supplementary oxygen at 15 litres per minute. Remember that a pulse oximeter may give a false high reading as it measures carbon dioxide in the blood in the same way it measures oxygen.

NOTE:
Carbon Monoxide is a flammable gas and as such represents a flammable atmosphere. Defibrillation must not be carried out indoors with a suspected carbon monoxide patient.

Heat Illness

Extremes of heat can have significant and detrimental effect on how the body functions and heat can affect our ability to function both physically and mentally. A high core body temperature can quickly become a life threatening condition and must be dealt with quickly. Normal body temperature for a healthy adult generally sits somewhere between 36.5° and 37.5°.

Heat Exhaustion

The signs and symptoms of heat exhaustion include:

- Temperature up to 40°C;
- Heart rate ≥ 100 per minute;
- Breathing fast and shallow;
- Low BP;
- Fatigue;
- Headache;
- Nausea and vomiting;
- Abdominal cramps, and/or
- Disorientation.

Heat Stroke

Heat stroke is a life threatening condition caused by a severe disruption of the body's thermoregulatory system. Symptoms include:

- Temperature > 40°C.
- Rapid heart rate.
- Constricted pupils.
- Dehydration.
- Pale and sweaty skin.
- Tremors.
- Acute confusion.
- Convulsions.
- Delirium or possible coma.

Management

Take a full set of observations including core body temperature. Readings from tympanic thermometers should not be relied on in isolation, and other signs and symptoms should be taken into account.

A rule of thumb when it comes to extremes of temperature is to cool quickly and warm slowly, so when your patient is hypothermic you warm them up at a slow and steady rate, when they are too warm you cool them quickly.

One of the most effective ways of reducing the core body temperature is radial cooling, which is often used by fire and rescue services to reduce the core body temperature of breathing apparatus wearers who have been working in temperatures of more than 100 degrees Celsius.

Radial cooling involves placing the wrists in cool water, cooling the blood in the radial arteries, which is then pumped around the body reducing the core temperature.

Dementia

As with COPD, dementia is an umbrella term to describe a range of conditions. These conditions are progressive ones that affect the brain (Dementia UK, 2019). There are over 200 subtypes with the five most common being Alzheimer's disease, vascular dementia, dementia with Lewy bodies, frontotemporal dementia and mixed dementia (Dementia UK, 2019).

Dementia affects the passage of messages throughout the brain by damaging the nerve cells. When these messages can no longer be passed effectively, the way the body functions can be affected.

People with dementia may become reliant on their long-term memory; this may mean that they relate things from the present as if they were in the past, or get complete strangers mixed up with close relatives. This can be extremely confusing. This confusion can lead to mood swing, and be extremely frightening for the individual.

Dementia is not simply about memory loss, it can affect the way a person thinks or behaves; it can affect the way they feel. Behavioural changes linked to dementia can include agitated behaviour, a loss of inhibitions where the sufferer acts in ways that would normally be seen as inappropriate, and repetitive questioning.

When dealing with a patient who has dementia it is important to listen, not to interrupt, and be patient. They may repeat questions, don't say things like "I have already told you" or "like I said earlier", simply repeat the information as if it's the first time the question has been asked.

When speaking, speak in a calm and relaxed manner, don't shout or speak loudly. Continually explain what is happening, who you are and why you are there.

Mental Health

Mental health issues can affect anyone, and even those who appear outwardly confident and happy may be fighting a battle that nobody knows about. Some people see it as a weakness and worry what others may think if they find out, this leads to them bottling things up and even trying to convince themselves that they do not have a problem.

The problem with trying to fight the battle yourself is that often it becomes too much, making the problem worse, and you shouldn't underestimate how difficult it can be to battle against your own thoughts and feelings, no matter how irrational they may seem to others.

We live in a world where things seem to move at an incredible pace, there are financial pressures; pressure to succeed; pressure from social media to act in a certain way or have certain look. This is not necessarily always the reason that people suffer from mental health issues, but it certainly does not help.

You wouldn't tell someone with a broken leg to pull themselves together or get a grip would you? It feels like an overused expression, but it is still relevant. Just because you cannot see an illness does not mean it isn't there.

Obsessive Compulsive Disorder

The common misconception about obsessive-compulsive disorder (OCD) is that it is all about liking things ordered and tidy and having the urge to straighten a wonky picture or line everything up on your desk at work.

OCD sufferers have obsessive thoughts that are unwanted and unpleasant; these thoughts enter the mind and can cause feelings of anxiety or unease. In response to these thoughts the sufferer often has compulsions to carry out certain acts that temporarily relieve the unpleasant feelings.

Anxiety

Everybody suffers from feelings of anxiety from time to time; exams, job interviews, and issues such as financial problems can all cause a person to feel anxious, and these feelings are completely normal.

A person suffering from an anxiety disorder has difficulty in controlling these feelings and they can become persistent, affecting the individual's day to day life. Anxiety disorders may cause the sufferer to catastrophise i.e. come up with the worst possible consequences resulting from an action or situation, no matter how illogical these seem to anyone else, they can seem like a very real possibility to the anxiety sufferer.

Depression

As with feelings of anxiety, feeling down or unhappy for a few days is quite common and is a perfectly normal response to an unhappy event. Genuine depression occurs when these feelings last for months rather than days.

Unfortunately, some people do not see depression as a real illness, but depression is not something that someone can simply snap out of.

Handover

The passage of information as a patient makes their journey from the scene to the hospital, then the surgeons table is vital, and if handovers are not clear and concise, the risk is that it becomes a bit like Chinese whispers.

During a handover there only one voice should be heard, it can be easy to miss a vital piece of information when people are talking in the background; do not be afraid to ask for silence. The information given should be passed over in a structured manner; it should be clear and concise an unnecessary talk should be avoided.

Trauma Handover	
N	Always use the patient's **name**
A	**Age**
T	**Time** of injury (If known) may be approximate
M	**Mechanism** of injury
I	**Injuries** found or suspected
S	**Signs** and **Symptoms**
T	**Treatments** given

Table 21 - NATMIST

Welfare

We all feel physically drained from time to time, and it's no different with our mental health, constant exposure to stress can lead to us becoming mentally drained. Struggling with your mental health does not mean that you are bad at your job, and it doesn't make you less of a person. We all have our stress tolerance limits, and sometimes when we reach or exceed them we need to reach out and get a little help, after all, you would seek help if you broke your leg, so why should mental health issues be any different?

The welfare of responders should be a primary concern for the trust for whom they respond, it should also be top of the priority list for the responder themselves, and that should include monitoring the welfare of others at the scene and within their team.

Responding to medical emergencies can be extremely stressful and can significantly affect mental health. Issues can arise following an accumulation of stressful or upsetting events, or they can result from a single incident and anyone can be affected. As a responder you should look for signs that you yourself, or other members of your team are struggling, and not just afterwards, looking for these signs during an incident is equally as important.

There are many sources of help available ranging from helplines and websites to counsellors through the NHS or private practitioners. It can also be helpful speaking to fellow responders, who will have an idea of what you face on a daily basis.

We all feel physically drained from time to time, and it's no different with our mental health, constant exposure to stress can lead to us becoming mentally drained. Struggling with your mental health does not mean that you are bad at your job, and it doesn't make you less of a person. We all have our stress tolerance limits, and sometimes when we reach or exceed them we need to reach out and get a little help, after all, you would seek help if you broke your leg, so why should mental health issues be any different?

Checklists

Despite what anyone may have told you, checklists are not cheating. As a CFR you may well have another profession, and a busy home life; remembering everything about everything can be difficult even if you haven't. In order to avoid mistakes, the airline industry provides its pilots with checklists which outline the procedures for known emergency events and pre-flight checks.

The great thing with checklists is that they can prevent the user from missing vital steps which is particularly important when flying an aircraft, and equally as important when you are attending to a patient; I am absolutely certain that if I was a patient, I would rather see the responder that came to my aid working through a checklist and being thorough, than missing something important that may affect my treatment.

Pharmacology

This section covers some of the more common medications that can be administered by CFR's and some of the more common medications you may come across as a CFR. Some medications, such as GTN sprays and asthma inhalers can be self-administered by the patient, but these must be their own prescribed medications. Others such as aspirin may be given by the responder, provided this is something that falls within their scope of practice.

IMPORTANT

Never give the patient any medications that you have not been trained to administer and for those that you can administer, always follow administration guidelines provided by your trust!

Aspirin

Aspirin is administered to help prevent clotting, and to reduce pain and temperature. It comes in 300mg dispersible tablets. The maximum dose given should be 1 x 300mg tablet.

The contra-indications for aspirin (or reasons not to give it) are:

- The patient has a known aspirin allergy;
- Haemophilia or a blood clotting disorder;
- Active gastrointestinal bleeding, or
- Severe hepatic disease.

Aspirin shouldn't be given to children under 16.

Aspirin is sometimes given to patients who we suspect are having heart attacks. In this case the aspirin acts as an anti-platelet medication and helps to reduce clotting, hopefully increasing blood flow to the heart.

Entonox

Entonox is an inhaled gas used for moderate to severe pain or labour pain. It is self-administered by the patient as required, via a mouthpiece or facemask. The side effects with Entonox are minimal.

The contra-indications for Entonox are:

- Patients with decompression sickness (the bends);
- Suspected pneumothorax/tension pneumothorax;
- Severe head injury with reduced level of consciousness;
- Violently disturbed psychiatric patients, or
- Recent eye operation with gas insufflation of the orbit.

Caution is advised when considering Entonox for patients at risk of having a pneumothorax, pneumomediastinum and/or a pneumoperitoneum (e.g. polytrauma, penetrating torso injury).

Oxygen

When the levels of oxygen in our patient's blood fall below normal levels i.e. 94 to 98 percent normally and 88 to 92 percent for a patient with COPD, we can administer supplementary oxygen in order to try and bring their oxygen levels back up.

The potential side effects of supplementary oxygen are that it can be drying and irritating to mucous membranes over time, and in patients with COPD there is a risk that even moderately high doses of inspired oxygen can produce increased carbon dioxide levels which may cause respiratory depression, and this may lead to respiratory arrest.

The only contra-indication for the use of supplementary oxygen is that it shouldn't be used in explosive atmospheres, and it should be remembered that oxygen increases fire risk.

When using a defibrillator, oxygen **MUST** be removed **PRIOR** to administering a shock.

Dextrose Gel

The route of administration for dextrose gel is buccal, which means that it is administered orally by applying to the inside of the cheek. The obvious contra-indication here is the patient who has a reduced level of consciousness, as the risk of choking or aspiration is high. Therefore the gel should only be given to patients with sufficient levels of consciousness.

After each dose the patient's blood glucose levels should be taken, and if necessary repeat doses can be given.

Communication

The communication of information in patient care, whether written or verbal, is vital in ensuring that your patient gets the right care in a timely manner. Communication should be concise, sticking to the facts of the case and should be passed from one individual to another, when you get several people trying to speak at the same time it is easy to miss a piece of risk critical information, and when the information comes from more than one source it can be conflicting.

To avoid confusion when spelling words out to others, particularly when communicating via radio the NATO phonetic alphabet should be used. Accents, particularly my broad Lancastrian accent, can cause issues as well and the use of the phonetic alphabet alleviates this issue.

NATO Phonetic Alphabet							
A	Alpha	**B**	Bravo	**C**	Charlie	**D**	Delta
E	Echo	**F**	Foxtrot	**G**	Golf	**H**	Hotel
I	Indigo	**J**	Juliet	**K**	Kilo	**L**	Lima
M	Mike	**N**	November	**O**	Oscar	**P**	Papa
Q	Quebec	**R**	Romeo	**S**	Sierra	**T**	Tango
U	Uniform	**V**	Victor	**W**	Whiskey	**X**	X-Ray
Y	Yankee	**Z**	Zulu				

Table 22 - NATO Phonetic Alphabet

Common Abbreviations			
AAA	Abdominal Aortic Aneurysm	**AED**	Automated External Defibrillator
AF	Atrial Fibrillation	**ALS**	Advanced Life Support
APLS	Advance Paediatric Life Support	**ATLS**	Advanced Trauma Life Support
AV	Atrioventricular	**BLS**	Basic Life Support
COPD	Chronic Obstructive Pulmonary Disease	**CPR**	Cardiopulmonary Resuscitation
CSF	Cerebrospinal Fluid	**CVA**	Cerebrovascular Accident
DKA	Diabetic Ketoacidosis	**DNR**	Do not Resuscitate
DVT	Deep Vein Thrombosis	**ECG**	Electrocardiogram
ET	Endotracheal	**GTN**	Glycerol Trinitrate
GCS	Glasgow Coma Scale	**HEMS**	Helicopter Emergency Medical Service
ICP	Intercranial Pressure	**IHD**	Ischaemic Heart Disease
IM	Intramuscular	**IV**	Intravenous

LMA	Laryngeal Mask Airway	**MAP**	Mean Arterial Pressure
MI	Myocardial Infarction	**NSAID**	Non-Steroidal Anti Inflammatory Drug
PE	Pulmonary Embolism	**PEA**	Pulseless Electrical Activity
PHTLS	Pre-hospital Trauma Life Support	**PR**	Per Rectum
RSI	Rapid Sequence Induction	**SAH**	Subarachnoid Haemorrhage
SC	Subcutaneous	**SVT**	Supra Ventricular Tachycardia
TIA	Transient Ischaemic Attack	**UTI**	Urinary Tract Infection
VF	Ventricular Fibrillation	**VT**	Ventricular Tachycardia

Table 23 - Common Abbreviations

Medical Terminology

Medical terms can be confusing, sometimes it is possible to figure out the meaning by splitting up the word such as haemothorax i.e. haemo relating to blood and thorax being the chest cavity, hence a haemothorax is blood in the chest cavity; anything with hypo in it refers to low and hyper relates to high and so on.

Directional Words	
Anterior	Front - (The kneecap is on the Anterior side of the leg)
Distal	Away from - (The foot is at the distal end of the leg)
Inferior	Lower/Below – (Below the waistline)
Lateral	Side - (Sides of the body, the little toe is at the lateral side of the foot)
Medial	Middle of the body
Posterior	Back of the body
Proximal	Close to (proximal end of the humerus attaches to the shoulder)
Superior	Above - (Above the waistline)
Ventral	Front, belly
Unilateral	On one side of the body only

Bilateral	Both sides of the body

Other Health Conditions

As a CFR you will come across patients with a range of health conditions that may or may not be related to the purpose of the emergency call. The purpose of this section is to introduce these conditions.

Pneumonia

Pneumonia is an infection of the lung tissue that causes the air sacs in the lungs to fill with fluid and become inflamed which prevents them from working properly.

Possible Symptoms of Pneumonia:

- New cough;
- Bringing up phlegm;
- Fever;
- Breathlessness or difficulty breathing;
- Chest pain or discomfort.

Crohn's Disease

Crohn's is a lifelong condition that affects the digestive system; it causes inflammation, most commonly in the small intestine and symptoms such as:

- Abdominal pain;
- Diarrhoea;
- Tiredness;
- Weight loss.

Multiple Sclerosis

Multiple Sclerosis (MS) affects the nervous system and prevents signals from being sent around the body properly. The word sclerosis means scarring and in MS scar tissue forms in many (or multiple) places around the nervous system.

Motor Neurone Disease

In Motor Neurone Disease (MND) the nerves that control the muscles used for breathing, swallowing, Speaking and moving gradually deteriorate preventing signals from the brain from reaching the muscles. MND is also known as amyotrophic lateral sclerosis (ALS).

Lyme Disease

Lyme disease is spread by bites from infected ticks found in long grass and woodlands. A tick is an arachnid typically between 2 and 5mm long. There are approximately 2000 – 3000 cases of Lyme disease diagnosed in England and Wales each year.

Commonly the disease causes flu like symptoms and an expanding bullseye rash. Other symptoms include:

- Neck stiffness;
- Nausea;
- Digestive issues.

If left untreated the disease can lead to pain and swelling in the joints, nervous systems issues, memory issues, headaches and migraines, heart problems, vertigo and dizziness, anxiety and depression.

Pancreatitis

Acute pancreatitis occurs when the pancreas becomes inflamed and is most commonly caused by gallstones or alcohol. Gallstones are hard pieces of material that form in the gallbladder.

The symptoms of pancreatitis include:

- A severe dull pain around the top of the stomach that develops suddenly.
- Nausea.
- Indigestion.
- Diarrhoea.
- Fever (temperature above 38°C).

- Jaundice.
- Tenderness in the abdomen.

Chronic pancreatitis occurs when the condition does not get better over time.

Parkinson's Disease

In Parkinson's disease the body does not produce enough of a chemical known as dopamine. Dopamine helps to control the muscles. The disease gets progressively worse over time and the rate at which it gets worse varies from person to person.

The most well-known symptom of Parkinson's is a tremor (shaking); other symptoms may include:

- Changes in the way the patient walks;
- Stiffness;
- Moving slower;
- Balance problems.

Leptospirosis

Leptospirosis, also known as Weil's disease is spread in the urine of infected animals, most commonly rats, mice, cows, pigs and dogs, and can be picked up in contaminated water courses, soil or blood from infected animals.

Symptoms include:

- Headache;
- Nausea and vomiting;
- Fever;
- Aching muscles and joints;
- Red eyes, an/or
- Loss of appetite.

References

BHF, 2014. *Policy Statement: Creating a Nation of Lifesavers,* London: British Heart Foundation.

BHF, 2019. *British Heart Foundation.* [Online]
Available at:
https://www.bhf.org.uk/informationsupport/conditions/heart-failure
[Accessed 7 November 2019].

Cecconi, M. et al., 2014. Consensus on circulatory shock and hemodynamic monitoring. Task force of the European Society of Intensive Care Medicine. *Intensive Care Medicine,* Issue 40, pp. 1795-1815.

Cox, D., 2017. *The Guardian: Health and Wellbeing.* [Online]
Available at:
https://www.theguardian.com/lifeandstyle/2017/sep/18/sepsis-the-truth-about-this-hidden-killer
[Accessed 24 September 2019].

Dementia UK, 2019. *Dementia UK.* [Online]
Available at: https://www.dementiauk.org/get-support/diagnosis-and-next-steps/what-is-dementia/?gclid=Cj0KCQjwuNbsBRC-ARIsAAzITuf9ewE2SslIMIUlSdFIeT7cCdi2kQCxfea66FSBruRCLc3DFZyFLYkaApoXEALw_wcB
[Accessed 3 October 2019].

FPHC, 2017. *Faculty of Pre-Hospital Care.* [Online]
[Accessed 18 December 2019].

NHS, 2017. *england.nhs.uk: our work.* [Online]
Available at: https://www.england.nhs.uk/ourwork/clinical-policy/sepsis/nationalearlywarningscore/
[Accessed 10 January 2020].

NHS, 2017. *NHS: Conditions.* [Online]
Available at: https://www.nhs.uk/conditions/epilepsy/
[Accessed 30 October 2019].

NICE, 2017. *NICE.* [Online]
Available at: https://cks.nice.org.uk/corneal-superficial-injury#!scenario
[Accessed 8 January 2020].

NICE, 2017. *NICE: Guidance.* [Online]
Available at:
https://www.nice.org.uk/guidance/ng51/chapter/Recommendations
[Accessed 17 January 2020].

NICE, 2018. *CKS.NICE.* [Online]
Available at: https://cks.nice.org.uk/carbon-monoxide-
poisoning#!diagnosisSub:1
[Accessed 12 November 2019].

Sepsis Trust, 2019. *Sepsis Trust: About Sepsis.* [Online]
Available at: https://sepsistrust.org/about/about-sepsis/
[Accessed 24 September 2019].

Other Books and Products Available from Rescue Guide

Emergency Response Field Guide

The emergency response field guide covers a large range of subjects relating to emergency response and is intended as an aide memoir for emergency responders.

Road Traffic Collisions: A Complete Guide

A complete guide to road traffic collisions covering pretty much every possible scenario you may come across as an emergency responder.

Scene Assessment Cards

A series of laminated pocket cards designed for emergency responders. Whatever you have been told, checklists are not cheating.

Vehicle Assessment Cards

Designed for road traffic collisions, these laminated cards take you through the process of vehicle related information gathering.

Medical Assessment Cards

A must for anyone who responds to medical emergencies, these laminated pocket cards cover patient assessment for the first responder.

For more information on Rescue Guide products visit
www.rescueguide.co.uk or email us at
publishing@rescueguide.co.uk

Follow us on Twitter: @Rescue_Guide

Facebook: https://www.facebook.com/Rescue-Guide

Printed in Great Britain
by Amazon